functional **OTOLOGY**
THE PRACTICE OF AUDIOLOGY

*f*unctional
∫OTOLOGY

THE PRACTICE OF
AUDIOLOGY

By MORRIS F. HELLER, M.D.
*Assistant Attending Otolaryngologist for Audiology, Chief of the
Audiology Clinic, The Mount Sinai Hospital, New York.*

with
Bernard M. Anderman, M.A.
and Ellis E. Singer, M.A.

SPRINGER SCIENCE+BUSINESS MEDIA, LLC

Copyright, 1955
Springer Science+Business Media New York
Originally published by Springer Publishing Company, Inc. in 1955
Softcover reprint of the hardcover 1st edition 1955

ISBN 978-3-662-39162-4   ISBN 978-3-662-40154-5 (eBook)
DOI 10.1007/978-3-662-40154-5

Library of Congress Catalog Card Number: 55-12218

PREFACE

This book has been written to show how the auditory functional examination and the rehabilitation of the acoustically handicapped patient can be integrated into otological practice. The scope and operation of large audiology centers of hospitals and universities are also considered.

The developments in audio-communication have been enormous during the past ten or twenty years. Similarly, the general interest in hearing has increased, as shown for instance by such terms as high fidelity an dstereophonic sound systems.

Specifically, industries and the military are concerned about injurious noise causing damage and loss of acoustic function; school systems and departments of health aim at early detection of hearing losses and at their correction. The problems connected with hearing are being investigated by otologists, pathologists, physiologists, psychologists, physicists, electro-engineers, audiologists, teachers of lip reading and speech, and teachers of the deaf.

These trends and their results are changing the practice of otology. The function of hearing is now probed and tested more easily, more exactly and more comprehensively than before. There is greater promise for alleviation of the handicap of deafness. The physician is expected to examine his patients with otic disease so that he can evaluate the pathology *and* the impairment of hearing which is the result of the pathology.

To make this book as widely useful as possible, effort has been made to take nothing for granted. The testing area is described as well as the equipment and how to use it and take care of it. Though technical proficiency and proven routines are shown to be necessary, the emphasis is on the judicious application and combination of tests and their relation to all other phases of the examination and diagnosis. The otologist must be able to determine whether a hearing loss is of organic causation or a manifestation of psychological problems of the patient; whether a child is deaf, or whether other organic factors exist that make it appear that a child cannot speak or hear. By showing how to produce detailed and meaningful audiograms of many kinds of hearing loss, their correct interpretation is explained also. The ultimate purpose of this book is to aid the physician and others participating in the field of functional otology in determining the rehabilitative requirements of the patient, how they shall be met, and who will institute the program of rehabilitation.

The indications for medical and surgical therapy are not included, as these are readily found in the available literature.

Two associates have contributed to this book, and I am happy to thank them for their participation. Bernard M. Anderman wrote the chapters on Speech Audiometry and on Hearing Aids which includes a timely description of transistor hearing aids. Ellis E. Singer wrote the important chapters on Voice and Speech Production, Speech Deviations in Conductive Deafness and in Perceptive Deafness, and on Auditory Rehabilitation.

MORRIS F. HELLER, M.D.

New York, N. Y.
October 1955

ACKNOWLEDGEMENTS:

For arrangements made with various publishing houses and authors whereby certain (copyrighted) material was permitted to be reprinted, acknowledgments are gratefully made.

To I. J. Hirsh and to Wayne University, publishers of Journal of Speech and Hearing Disorders, and to the McGraw-Hill Book Company, publishers of The Measurement of Hearing, for letting us reprint the Auditory Test Lists W-1, W-2, and W-22.

To the Annals Publishing Company for letting us reprint (1) the list of equipment and supplies, in Chapter 3, and the chronology of study and care, at the end of the book, both taken from a paper by Heller and Lindenberg published in the Annals of Otology, Rhinology and Laryngology; (2) portions of "Tinnitus aurium in normal hearing persons" by Heller and Bergman published also in the Annals.

To the American Medical Association for material taken from "Evaluation of deafness of non-organic origin" by Heller and Lindenberg, published in the A.M.A. Archives of Otolaryngology.

To the Bureau of Handicapped Children, Department of Health, New York City, for its "Recommended Standards for Audiology Centers" the substance of which forms the second chapter of this book.

CONTENTS

functional **OTOLOGY**
THE PRACTICE OF AUDIOLOGY

1

OFFICE TESTING AREA

The noise level of a quiet domestic dwelling is about 35 to 40 decibels. The noise level of a relatively quiet business office may vary from 40 to 50 decibels. In a noisier area the level may be as much as 70 decibels. Heavy industry, riveting, chipping, caulking, and drilling in compressed air will produce noise levels well in excess of 100 decibels.

It is apparent that testing people's hearing at different noise levels will result in obtaining different thresholds of hearing. Day in and day out we who have normal hearing modify our voice volume depending upon the loudness of the environmental masking noise above which we must talk in order to be heard. High ambient noise levels mask the hearing, and the hearing threshold of the moment is altered depending upon the masking level. When testing hearing, the ambient noise level should therefore be reduced so that it will not materially affect the test findings. An ambient noise level of less than 30 decibels can be discounted as a masking factor for clinical testing and can be obtained without too much constructional difficulties.

Although in ordinary daily living hearing is not performed in artificially created quiet surroundings, we can find the maximum acuity of an ear only under quiet and controlled conditions. If all the factors in testing are constant except the patients themselves, we have a stable starting point. In addition, the same patient may be tested at intervals over many years; if all external factors remain constant, the stability or changes in the test results will be of real significance.

Two adjoining rooms, each of modest size, are desirable; one for the patient and the other for the observer and the equipment. A cubicle for the patient is not as satisfactory. A one-way vision window, installed directly to the side of the seated patient and permitting a direct view by the tester is decidedly advantageous. Most patients are more relaxed when they think they are not being observed, and the patient's spontaneous behavior at times offers useful clues revealing his personality and reliability. The sound damped room in which the patient sits can be approximately 8' x 8' x 4'. This is large enough to permit pure tone audiometry with head phones, free field speech hearing testing, and hearing aid fitting. A somewhat larger room will allow space for testing infants and young children which requires additional equipment. These tests, such as galvanic skin response audiometry and peep show audiometry, can also be performed in an untreated room; generally, the clinical problem is to determine whether these little patients are severely deafened or their hearing is within near-normal values.

The Sound Treated Room

The walls of the sound-treated test room can be of cinder block or plaster to which is attached some material that effectively sound damps the room. There are several materials which satisfactorily attenuate noise.

The author built his own sound damped room with only

a little architectural advice and with the assistance of un-skilled labor. Strips of wood, 1" x 2" and 2" x 2", known as *furring*, were nailed to the walls, horizontally at the junction of the walls and the ceiling, vertically at the junction of adjoining walls. 2" x 2" strips were nailed low down on the walls, horizontally. By this means frames were formed in depth equal to the thickness of the attenuating material, which in this instance was fiber glass.

Fiber glass boards are available 48" x 24" x 2". They are light in weight and are easily cut with a knife or scissors. Gloves were worn when handling the board, as the glass spicules rub off and stick into the skin. The boards were affixed to the walls and ceiling within the wooden frames with appropriate adhesive paste, which can be purchased with the fiber glass.

An inexpensive cotton fabric which blended with the office decor was used to cover the fiber glass on the walls and ceiling. The fabric was stapled to the furring strips, covering all construction, except for outlets and window. Cut-outs in the walls were made for electrical oultets, for leads to and from the testing equipment and for a window, approximately 2' x 2'.

A free field speaker baffle, described in *Chapter 3*, was installed within this room during the course of construction. The baffle was attached to the ceiling about eight feet from the patient's position and the speaker was beamed directly at the patient. A portable corner baffle is suitable, also. The choice of baffle may be dictated by the available space in the room. The speaker should be installed within the baffle in such a manner that it can be removed for repairs without making it necessary to remove the cabinet. The cabinet was lined with fiber glass in order to dampen unwanted reflection of sound from the walls of the baffle.

The door also was treated with the fiber glass. Special

doors and their jambs are commercially available; these
have a sound seal along the bottom of the door, which automatically drops down when the door is closed and seals the
door and floor. Weather stripping attached to the edges of
the door produces an inexpensive but somewhat less effective
seal.

The floor may also be sound treated. The attenuating
material is laid on the floor and a metal grill placed over it.
Carpeting is used to cover the grill.

If the remainder of the office is generally quiet, a room
so constructed should have an ambient noise level of 30 decibels or less. The noise level should be measured after the
furniture has been put into the room.

To ventilate such a room without increasing the noise
level may present a problem. An induction and return ven-
tilating and cooling system is expensive and may be noisy.
The installation of air ducts requires additional openings
in the room which tend to nullify the effort made to obtain
sufficient dampening. If the room is about as large as previously described, ordinary electric fans which operate when
the room is vacant, though less than ideal, are serviceable.

The ambient decibel value of the room should be included in reports of the test findings. This is important
when tests are compared which were performed on one
patient at several different places.

The Equipment Room

The equipment room is immediately adjacent to the
sound treated room. The equipment itself is grouped about
the one-way vision window, so that the observer performing
the tests can manipulate the apparatus easily while observ-
ing the patient.

This room should be larger than the other as additional uses are made of it. Some of the equipment will be used during the class work of auditory rehabilitation. Classes consist of groups of 4 to 6 patients and a teacher.

This room need not be sound-treated. One of the advantages of such a "live" room is that during auditory training periods the patients will be listening with their hearing aids under environmental conditions more like those with which they are familiar. If patients learn to use hearing aids at low ambient levels, which is a more comfortable environment for hearing with amplification, they will be more distressed by the higher levels of the everyday "live" situations.

2

AUDIOLOGY CENTERS

Large audiology centers are usually affiliated with hospitals or universities, carry a heavy case load, and are concerned also with teaching and research programs. Such centers require an appreciable amount of space and construction. The following description of an audiology center is based on recommendations of the New York City Department of Health.*

The standards were developed, with the assistance of an advisory committee, as a guide for hospitals that are interested in developing audiology centers. Although the recommended standards relate to the care of children and youth, it is not intended that the audiology centers limit themselves to their care. The advisory committee was of the opinion that the "team method" is necessary in such centers, namely, that the professional personnel must be brought together and work together.

Functions of an Audiology Center

It aids in the education of the community regarding the prevention of hearing loss, by understanding the causes of

---

* Recommended Standards for Audiology Centers, Bureau of Handicapped Children, Helen M. Wallace, M.D., Director, Department of Health, New York City, 1953 (mimeographed).

hearing problems and the need for early detection, treatment, training and rehabilitation.

It provides services in which children and youth who have or are suspected of having defective hearing can be examined, diagnosed and treated.

It provides services for children and youth whose hearing loss necessitates special instruction and/or the use of a hearing aid.

Recommended Personnel. Patient-Personnel Ratios

A. Director

The Director or Coordinator of the auditory center, preferably full time, will serve as the administrator, responsible for the maintenance of a high quality of service and for the coordination of the work of each member of the staff. The director or coordinator should be a physician, preferably an otolaryngologist, or an audiologist. The latter must hold an Advanced Certificate in Hearing issued by the American Speech and Hearing Association (A.S.H.A.) or equivalent.

B. Medical Staff

(1) One or more qualified *otologists* for the complete otological evaluation of patients. One otologist should see no more than twelve patients per three-hour session.

(2) One or more qualified *pediatricians* for the complete pediatric evaluation of patients. One pediatrician should see no more than twelve patients per three-hour session.

(3) *Consultants* in the fields of neurology, orthodontia, orthopedic surgery, plastic surgery, psychiatry, etc. These should be readily available to the staff of the audiology center. Qualification: Diplomates of the respective specialty board or physicians who have the training and experience

necessary for admission to the examination of the respective boards.

C. Non-Medical Professional Staff

(1) A minimum of two full-time *audiologists,* each seeing an average of four to six patients a day. Qualification: Must meet the requirements for the Basic Certificate in Hearing issued by the A.S.H.A.

(2) A minimum of two *audiometric technicians,* each seeing an average of twenty patients per day. Qualifications: Must meet the requirements for the Basic Certificate in Hearing issued by the A.S.H.A.

(3) A minimum of two *hearing therapists,* one of whom should have had experience in the education of the deaf. Each therapist should see no more than twenty-five patients per day in individual and group therapy. Qualifications: Must meet the requirements for the Basic Certificate in Hearing issued by the A.S.H.A. plus the certification requirements set up by the Conference of Executives of the American Schools for the Deaf.

(4) A minimum of two *speech therapists,* each seeing no more than twenty-five patients per day in individual and group therapy. Qualifications: Must meet the requirements for the Basic Certificate in Speech issued by the A.S.H.A.

(5) A *psychologist.* The hospital should have a psychology department which meets professional standards. The psychologist assigned to the audiology center should be well-grounded in the problems arising from disorders of communication. Preferably, he should be trained in education of the handicapped child.

(6) At least one full-time *social worker.* The hospital should have a social service department which meets professional standards. Qualifications: The case worker should have a full graduate curriculum in social case work in an

accredited school of social work; he must be working under supervision of a social work supervisor or have previously worked two years in a social service department of acceptable standards in a medical setting under qualified supervision.

The supervisor must meet the same educational requirements as the caseworker and have a minimum of two years' full-time paid supervised casework experience in a social service department of acceptable standards in a medical setting. When responsibility for supervision of social casework is carried by a single person, the qualifications should be identical to those of a supervisor.

Recommended Physical Setup

An integrated unit should be provided for all facilities and services of the center, within a hospital which can furnish the recommended consultative services.

The center should be located in a quiet section of the hospital, away from any heavy machinery, main plumbings, etc. An adequate amount of space must be provided within the center which should be treated for sound absorption and exclusion in its entirety.

Rooms Necessary

(1) *Reception area and waiting space* (30' x 20')

(2) *Office for director or coordinator* (10' x 15')

(3) *Office for social worker* (10' x 10')

(4) *Office for psychologist* (10' x 10')

(5) *Playroom,* adequately equipped (20' x 20')

(6) *Auditory training rooms* (two). Small room for individual training; large room for group training (10' x 10' and 10' x 20').

(7) *Speech therapy rooms* (two). Small room for individual training; large room for group training. Both rooms should have running water. (10' x 10' and 10' x 20').

(8) *Office for general personnel.* For record keeping, record filing and staff conferences. (20' x 10')

(9) *Medical examination rooms.* Their number will depend on the case load of patients and on the number of physicians assigned to the center. Each room should have running water and suction.

(10) *Sound-proofed section.* Must be thoroughly treated for sound absorption and transmission; special doors, no windows; air conditioning (acoustically treated) desirable. Noise level of not more than 30 decibels overall.

a. *Testing suites.* There should be two two-room testing suites, each consisting of a test room for the patient and a control room for the technician. (30' x 15')

b. *Audiometric testing rooms (two).* (10' x 5' each).

(11) *Ear mold laboratory.* Should have running water. (5' x 5').

(12) *Storage space.* In general area and sound-proofed section.

(13) *Electronics workshop.* This may be a part of the general instrument repair shop of the hospital.

Recommended Minimum Equipment

A. *Basic Audiometric Testing Rooms*

One basic two-channel audiometer in each room.

B. *Auditory Training Rooms*

(1) Group equipment for large room; individual equipment for small room; mirror in each room.

(2) One motion picture projector.

C. *Speech therapy rooms*

(1) For each room: full length mirror; relaxation table; orthopedic chair.

(2) One tape recorder.

D. *Sound-proofed Section*

(1) *For each two-room testing suite*: One hearing evaluation assembly consisting of (a) two channel units, one for speech, one for noise. (b) Outputs through any combination of head phones and/or through speaker, for one or both channels. The maximum output through phones should be 100 decibels or more, and for speaker 85 decibels.

(2) *For each (advanced) audiometric testing room*: Two-channel pure tone audiometer (advanced clinical audiometer).

E. *General*

Table model hearing aids should be provided in each room of the center except the audiometric testing rooms and auditory training rooms.

General Policies

Evaluation of Patient

Each patient seen in the center should have audiometric testing with an individual pure-tone audiometer. If any patient shows, on the basis of an audiometric test, a loss of 20 decibels or more in any two frequencies in either ear, the patient would then:

(1) Receive a complete evaluation by the otologist.

(2) Receive a complete evaluation by the pediatrician

unless a recent pediatric evaluation report is sent to the center.

(3) Receive a complete pure-tone and speech audiometric evaluation (threshold and supra threshold) by the audiologist.

(4) Receive a speech evaluation.

(5) Receive a psychological evaluation if indicated.

(6) If indicated, would be seen by any of the medical specialists (neurologist, orthodontist, orthopedic surgeon, plastic surgeon, psychiatrist, etc.).

(7) The findings of the diagnostic work-up and its evaluation are then presented at the staff conference of the professional personnel, at which time a decision on the plan for treatment is decided on for the patient, including medical treatment, surgical treatment and/or auditory rehabilitation.

(8) After the plan has been made the patient would be seen by the social worker.

Treatment and Rehabilitation

The services provided might be (1) *Medical.* (2) *Nonmedical*: Speech reading; speech therapy; auditory training; psychological guidance; selection, fitting and instruction in use of hearing aids; parent guidance; social casework; liaison with referral to schools and (for youths 14 years and over who require it) to the appropriate vocational guidance agency.

Staff Conferences

All the professional personnel of the center should meet periodically, preferably every week. These conferences should include not only a review of individual patients but also of problems in the operation of the services of the center and of advances in the field.

Records and Statistics

Complete records of patients should be maintained by the center. The center should routinely provide copies of the records (1) to the school which the child is attending; (2) to any referring physician. Statistics should be kept of all patients to whom casework services have been given.

Appointments

Patients should be seen in the center by appointment only, except in the case of an emergency. The center should provide a method of follow-up for those patients who do not keep their appointment.

3

EQUIPMENT

Equipment suggests many things—apparatus as well as their quality, quantity, reliability, versatility. Equipment implies one's ingenuity and ability to use the units and component parts effectively, to recognize when they are operating properly and when they are defective. Maintaining the equipment in satisfactory working order may require the skill of a competent audio engineer familiar with this specialized field.

The equipment consists of two basic units, one for pure tone testing and the other for speech hearing testing. Other apparatus contribute their share so that these tests can be accomplished properly and accurately.

It is not imperative that all the equipment be obtained at one time. A pure tone two channel audiometer can be purchased to which the subsidiary components can be added later. A turn table or tape player for speech hearing testing by phones can be added, and subsequently free field testing equipment. Units such as the peep show and psychogalvanometer and accessory elements may be selected as needed.

The Audiometer

Prior to the first quarter of the twentieth century, hearing tests were performed with percussion, string and wind instruments, among them tuning forks, monochord, Galton whistle, and with the spoken and whispered voice. The precision of tests was limited. The audiometer was introduced as a tool which could be relied upon to emit acoustic signals at frequencies and intensities which could be selected and reproduced at will.

Advantages of the audiometer are: any frequency within the limitations of the audiometer can be reproduced as often as needed for any one patient and from patient to patient. Any intensity within the limits of the audiometer can also be reproduced as frequently as necessary, within clinical tolerances. The signal can be emitted at an intensity for as long a duration as is desired. The signal can be interrupted and reproduced as frequently as need be. Records can be made of the findings of the tests, which are charted in symbolic language and numerical values. These are permanent records, and reasonably accurate comparisons with other similar tests can be made.

Most audiometers are rather expensive, heavy, usually bulky, and require some maintenance. Recently, small portable audiometers, light in weight, have been manufactured. Audiometers require care and attention, and at times they must be repaired. At such times one loses the services of this equipment. Air conduction receivers and bone conductors are easily damaged by rough handling. The cords may wear and break. Such units are susceptible to the hazards of all electric audio apparatus.

Clinical audiometers are designed for practical daily use. These audiometers have sufficient range of frequencies and intensities so that a reasonable evaluation of hearing can be obtained.

Some audiometers are of the discrete frequency type, others are sweep frequency audiometers. The discrete frequency type contains a frequency selector by which only several individual frequencies can be selected and no others. Sweep frequency audiometers are built so that the frequency selector can be rotated uninterruptedly, sweeping from the lowest to the highest frequency of the instrument. However, except for the major frequencies, the calibration of these audiometers is not necessarily accurate, so that sweep frequency audiometers offer only little more flexibility or latitude than the others.

The frequencies incorporated in audiometers vary only slightly amongst the several different makes of instruments. These frequencies are: 128 (125) cycles per second, 256 (250) cps, 512 (500) cps, 1024 (1000) cps, 2048 (2000) cps, 4096 (4000) cps, 8192 (8000) cps, 9747 (10000) cps. Some discrete frequency audiometers also include frequencies of 3000 cps, 5000 cps, and 6000 cps.

The audiometric mensuration is the decibel,* which allows for the easy handling of large numbers.

The tone produced by the audiometer can be interrupted

---

* The decibel is a tenth of a bel. It is a dimensionless, logarithmic unit expressing the ratio of two amounts of power. The expression of the intensity of a sound level is meaningful only when it is related to a reference intensity. Mathematically the ratio is described as follows:

$$\text{decibel level} = 10 \log_{10} \frac{I_1}{I_2}$$

where I_1 is the intensity under consideration at any moment, and I_2 is the basic reference intensity. A sound which has ten times the power of that of the reference is 10 decibels above the reference. If I_1 is 100 times the power of the reference I_2, the logarithm of their ratio, 100, is 2; and the number of decibels is $10 \times 2 = 20$ decibels. Each successive ten-fold increase in acoustic power indicates a corresponding addition of 10 decibels.

In most sound measurements, the reference sound intensity has been established as the quantity of 10^{-16} watts per square centimeter. This factor is related to the more familiar reference of acoustic pressure at 0.0002 dynes per square centimeter. These values are less than those of minimal physiological acoustic awareness.

Clinically, in testing hearing, the average sensitivity values of young adult normal ears for pure tones of the audiometric spectrum is taken to be 0 decibels. This value is above the acoustic zero reference intensity of 0.0002 dynes per square centimeter.

and recalled by the operation of an interrupter switch. The spring type of interrupter key must be held in the "off" position or the attenuator must be turned down to prevent the signal from reaching the receiver and be heard. Some interrupter keys have another position, which is not activated by a spring and the key must be manually operated to either "on" or "off."

The electrical energy output of the audiometer is converted into sound by the air conduction receiver or bone conductor just as a telephone receiver converts electrical energy into sound. Contemporary bone conductors lack the fidelity of air conduction receivers, especially at the highest frequencies. More electrical energy is required to activate the bone conductor and have the signal heard through the skull. For this reason audiometer attenuators are calibrated both for air conduction audiometry and for bone conduction audiometry. Some audiometers have two sets of numbers on the attenuator dial in contrasting colors indicating the decibel scale, one scale for air conduction and the other scale for bone conduction. Some earlier audiometers have a metal ring appropriately inscribed which is fitted over the air conduction numerals when bone conduction tests are performed. The bone conduction thresholds are read on the metal ring scale.

The internal design of audiometers consists of a chassis on which is mounted an audio signal generator and amplifier. This includes an attenuator (volume), frequency selector (tone), vacuum tubes, transformers, resistors, condensers, filters and other components. The function is such that an oscillating vacuum tube whose frequency is controlled by a network of resistors, capacitors, and inductors produces an alternating current which, when amplified by other vacuum tubes, ultimately is transformed into sound by the receiver.

The frequency of the alternating current can be selected; only one frequency is generated at a given moment. The amplitude of each frequency is controlled by the attenuator. The net results, in subjective terms, are that various tones can be heard and their loudness can be altered, increased and decreased.

In audio circuits adventitious sounds may occur from any defective component, or from switch noises, or with changes during the movements of the attenuator or frequency selector. If adventitious sounds are detected, there is indication of some defect in the audiometer which should be corrected.

The earlier audiometers consisted of a single output circuit, with one receiver. Such single channel audiometers are still available and usually are less expensive than two channel instruments. The two channel audiometers are more flexible for the administration of the various tests and offer advantages not obtainable in single channel units. Dual systems simplify the administration of such techniques as masking, recruitment testing, and Stenger audiometry. Two channel audiometers usually incorporate one frequency selector and two attenuators; each attenuator controls its own receiver.

Masking Apparatus

Masking is a method whereby the acoustic function of an ear can be removed from participating in hearing sound stimuli which are presented to the other ear. The objective of masking is to occlude the ear not being tested, just as the ophthalmologist occludes an eye he wishes to remove from the visual testing situation by covering it. It is apparent that merely covering an ear will not successfully prevent it from being aware of acoustic stimuli in the environment if the intensities of the stimuli are great enough.

The transmission of intensities greater than 50 decibels may be airborne around the skull and through the skull by bone conduction, vibrating the skull and with it both cochleae.

Many masking devices have been used from time to time. A widely known instrument is the Barany alarm apparatus. The masking noise produced by the Barany is composed almost entirely of low frequencies, the instrument vibrates excessively and it cannot be calibrated.

An audio system with its receiver can be assembled to produce a noise which serves for masking. Either of two masking noises is used in audiometry: *white* noise or *saw tooth* noise. White noise is composed of the audible frequencies emitted with uniform electrical energy. The term *white* is derived from a comparison to white light, which includes all the visual frequencies. Saw tooth noise contains only certain frequencies, in descending amplitudes.

An audio noise generator may be an independent unit, or may be physically contained within the audiometer. The masking intensity, controlled by its own attenuator, can be measured in decibels.

Speech Hearing Equipment

In order to measure the patient's ability to hear speech and to understand speech, additional equipment and selected speech material are required. Speech reception threshold tests and speech discrimination tests are performed with ear phones and with a free field speaker. The phones are required so that the speech hearing function of each ear can be measured individually. The free field speaker is necessary for hearing aid fittings, whereby measurements are made both of the unaided hearing and whatever improvement is obtained by means of the amplification of a hearing aid.

The units for speech hearing testing are composed of: (1) a speech reproducer, either phonograph disc player or magnetic tape reproducer; (2) recorded lists on disc or tape of spondaic words (*See Chapter 11*) and phonetically balanced words; (3) an audiometer with an input for the disc player or tape reproducer.

For these tests the speech stimuli replace the pure tone stimuli of the audiometer. The speech testing equipment is wired into the audiometer, and with selection of the proper circuits by a switch, speech from the reproducing equipment reaches the audiometer phone and is heard by the patient. The intensity of the speech is controlled by the attenuator of the audiometer, as in pure tone audiometry. The techniques of obtaining speech reception thresholds and speech discrimination scores are described in *Chapter 11*, Speech Audiometry.

A microphone for live voice is inserted into the circuit, essentially paralleling the circuit of the reproducing unit. Again, selecting the microphone circuit by a switch, the tester can make use of his own voice instead of recorded speech. A V-U meter for monitoring (see next page) is incorporated in the microphone circuit.

Free Field Equipment

The loud-speaker for free field testing is placed in the sound damped room, six to eight feet from the patient's position. The loud-speaker's response curve—fidelity—is important. The loud-speaker, of 12-inch to 15-inch diameter, must be contained in a suitable cabinet; the bass reflex or infinite baffle are common types. These cabinets are of the kind used in high fidelity radio and phonograph systems.

The purpose of the baffle is to prevent the back waves of

the loud-speaker's diaphragm from cancelling its front waves. The signals from the speaker are directed forward from the front of the speaker cone and also from its other surfaces. These latter sounds are reflected from the walls of the speaker cabinet and the walls of the room unless these are treated with acoustic damping material.

Speakers of this size and for this purpose are usually of the permanent magnetic type and require an amplifier to drive them. The amplifier has its own volume control. If no calibrated attenuator is in this amplifying circuit one must be inserted in the circuit in order that the tester will be able to deliver the material in measured amounts. The amplifier can be wired through the audiometer circuit, and the audiometer attenuator is then relied upon.

With a unit consisting of amplifier and speaker, stimulus from a sound source can be delivered to the patient. These sources are the pure tones of the audiometer, masking noise, recorded speech material from disc players and magnetic tape recorder-players, and live voice spoken into a microphone.

Basically this is an annunciator system in which the several components are of high fidelity and in proper calibration designed to serve the needs of testing hearing for speech reception and speech discrimination.

Volume Unit Meter

A V-U *(volume unit)* meter should be included in the live voice circuit. This is a small meter the needle of which is moved when speech or any other sound energy enters the microphone. The meter permits calibration of voice and speech; as one speaks into the microphone he can read on the meter the levels to which his voice volume drives the needle.

With experience one can speak into the microphone and keep one's speech volume to a fairly uniform level. With this accomplished the intensity of the speech will then be controlled by the attenuator of the audiometer or amplifier.

The monitored live voice technique is more effective when testing children and those adults who cannot easily adapt themselves to the machine-like rate of recorded speech.

Talk Back Unit

Because the patient is alone in the sound-damped test room and because he must repeat aloud the words as he hears them during the speech hearing tests, there is need of another sound communication system whereby the tester can hear what the patient says. This talk-back system consists of a microphone, in the immediate vicinity of the patient, which is wired to a smaller amplifier unit and speaker in front of the tester permitting the observer to listen to the patient as he speaks. The amplifier has in addition to the speaker a phone receiver head set; the observer can listen either with the speaker or with the phones, selecting either by turning a switch. The talk-back unit is indispensable when speech hearing tests are performed. Additionally, as the tester has a microphone through which he can communicate with the patient, either by the free field speaker or through the patient's receivers, and also a talk-back system through which the patient can speak with the observer; the two can converse whenever necessary.

Hearing Aid Baffle

Hearing aid fittings can be performed somewhat on the order of a blindfold test. If the hearing aids with which the patient is fitted are not exposed to the patient's view he is less likely to venture an opinion about any of the aids by any preconceptions, or by what he may have heard about any one make of aid. If the patient does not know with which aid he is being fitted, he can make a comparison subjectively only on what and how he hears with the aids. He will not even know when his own aid is included during the fitting process.

A receptacle for the hearing aid consists of a baffle mounted behind the patient. This baffle consists of a wooden board about ten or twelve inches square, on which is attached some acoustic attenuating material such as an acoustic tile block. To this is fastened a small cloth pocket into which a hearing aid is inserted. The distance between this baffle and the patient's ear is somewhat less than the average length of a hearing aid cord, which permits the hearing aid receiver to be inserted into the patient's ear and the cord to be connected both to the receiver and to the hearing aid.

Furniture

The furniture within the sound treated room can be simple and of as few individual pieces as consistent with comfort. When changes are made in the furnishings in such a room the acoustic values of the room may be altered. A chair is needed for adults who are tested, and a table and smaller chair for children, who may object to being placed alone in a room and may want a parent to be in the room with them.

Psychogalvanic Skin Equipment

The equipment for performing psychogalvanic skin re-

sponse audiometry consists of an audiometer, a galvanometer, and an inductorium.* The inductorium is of the
type often used in physiology laboratories. It is composed of
two coils, of which the primary is energized by a dry cell
battery. The interrupter of the inductorium rapidly makes
and breaks the flow of current through the primary coil.
The induced current of the secondary coil, faradic current,
is used to shock the patient gently during the preliminary
conditioning period of the testing.

The galvanometer must be sensitive enough to detect
changes of electrical potentials in the skin. Both inductorium and galvanometer are commercially available in inexpensive battery operated models. They can also be obtained
with audiometers. The shelf life of batteries is reasonably
long; nevertheless, they may have deteriorated to a degree
to vitiate successful testing. Accordingly, battery energized
equipment should be inspected in advance of the performance of a test, in order that one may be assured that the
several units function satisfactorily.

Peep Show

Various "peep shows" have been described by their de-
signers. The purpose of the peep show is to entertain the
children, interest them in the test and condition them to
respond to the acoustic stimuli. One type of peep show consists of a cabinet whose dimensions are about 24" x 24" x16".

---

* Recently, vacuum tube electro-stimulators have been designed.
Apparatus are available also which combine the several components. A
stylus records the skin potential changes on a moving spool of paper. These
records do not show characteristics such as seen in electrocardiographs.
Accordingly the examiner must determine which 'curves' are responses due
to acoustic stimulation, distinguishing them from random traces. It is necessary to write notations on the graph paper as the test proceeds. Unfor-
tunately present equipment construction fails to make adequate provision
for this.

The front wall of the cabinet contains a window approximately 6" x 6". A small inexpensive turntable of about two revolutions per minute, such as those used in store window displays, is placed within the cabinet and operates from the house electric current. On the turntable are mounted small toys which will amuse children, such as tin soldiers and similar figures for the boys, and small dolls and dollhouse furniture for the girls. Within the cabinet a light socket is mounted, into which a small light bulb is inserted. Beneath the window on the front wall of the cabinet is an electric spring switch for the child to manipulate.

A separate component is a switch box; the switch itself can be a single-throw, double pole anticapacity switch. The wiring layouts of the switch box circuits (Fig. 1) are as follows: from the audiometer there extend to the input-legs on one side of the switch in the switch box the leads through

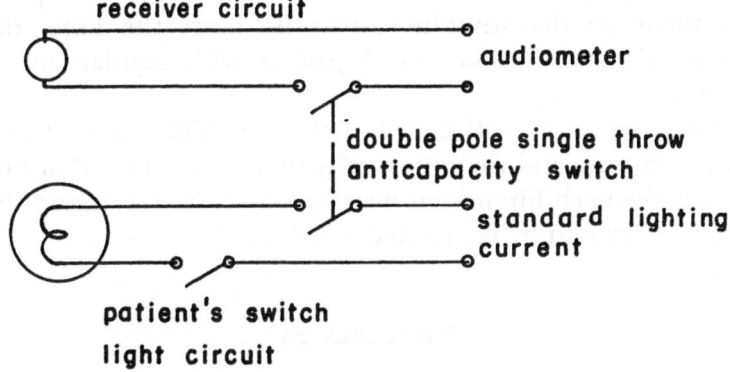

Fig. 1—Peep show audiometric and light circuits.

which the electrical energy of the tone stimulus flows; to other outgoing legs of this switch are attached the wire leads which connect either with the air conductor receiver, which is held to the child's ear, or to a free field speaker. Two other leads, from the house current, are attached to other independent legs of this same switch. The output of this second circuit is connected to the switch and light socket of the peep show. Accordingly, when the switch of the switch box is at the "on" position the tone from the audiometer is heard at the receiver, or speaker, and the current to the light bulb in the cabinet is interrupted only by the patient's switch on the cabinet. The patient is taught to push his peep show switch only when he hears the tone, and in so doing illuminates the interior of the cabinet so that the peep show is visible to him through the window. When the switch in the box is turned to "off" by the tester, both the tone and the light circuits are interrupted. If the child operates his own switch at this time the light cannot be turned on. The child becomes conditioned to activate his own switch only when he hears the tone. Once the child learns this sequence audiometry can be performed in an orderly manner for the several frequencies. Since the child does not know when the operator turns on the stimulus unless he hears the tone, the thresholds can be determined just as with regular audiometry.

The peep show will usually hold the child's interest and entertain him, and the test usually may be completed at one sitting. Some children soon become bored, however, and the test may have to be completed at a later date.

Noise-makers

Other sound producing apparatus used to test infants and little children are whistles, bells, musical triangles, toy "crickets" and others which the tester may select. A rough estimate of the frequencies of these various items and their intensities can be made.

Usually two observers are required when testing with

noise-makers; one observes the child and holds his attention, while the other stands behind the patient and activates the noise producers. A mentally healthy, normal-hearing, active child will respond when he hears these sounds, whereas a deaf child will remain unresponsive. A child may hear only some of these sounds but not all, and the observers will have obtained some evidence of the status of the infant's hearing. (*See Chapter 10*).

Ear Insert Supplies

The otologist should prepare the impression of the patient's auricle and meatus for the permanent ear insert. The insert which is clipped to the air conduction receiver of the hearing aid is inserted into the external auditory canal, as the hearing aid is worn. Each insert, as with dentures, requires individual fabrication.

A commercial laboratory which converts the impression of the canal and auricle into the permanent acrylic insert will supply the otologist with the necessary ingredients with which the original impression can be made.

Formerly plaster of Paris was used as the impression compound, but new synthetic materials have been developed which are easier to apply. The mix is prepared into a viscid mass which is inserted and molded to the contour of the auricle and meatus. The impression material is permitted to set and harden; it is removed from the ear, and sent to the laboratory. From this model the permanent insert is fabricated.

Because some inserts may be too long or have high spots, the otologist will need a small dental engine or bench engine and some small abrasive stones, buffers, and polishers in order to make minor changes in the configuration of the

acrylic insert. The laboratory or a dental associate can advise
the otologist when he purchases these supplies.

Auditory Training Unit

The instruction program in auditory training is designed
to teach patients to learn how to hear sounds and speech
artificially amplified by the audio system of the hearing aid.
Appropriate recorded material is presented by record player
or magnetic tape player through a loud-speaker, to which
the patients listen with the hearing aid. Phonograph records
can be cut with the environmental sounds of life recorded
on them. They can be similarly recorded on tape. Some of
these sounds are derived from horns, buzzers, bells, barking
dogs, telephone signals, running water, rustling of paper,
matches being struck, and others ad infinitum.

The audio equipment used for speech testing can be utilized during these lessons for listening purposes. An additional portable loud-speaker in its own cabinet can be added
to the amplifier circuit.

Additional Supplies

Demonstrations with skulls, anatomic pictures, and other
anatomical illustrations of the head can be used effectively
to help the patients understand the complexity of the otic
structures. Motion pictures are available illustrating in
simple diagrammatic form the otic anatomy and function.

With an interoffice telephone system connecting several
instruments, the patients can be taught to listen to phone
conversation with their hearing aids. Communal office telephones are available and the interoffice system can be
brought into service by push button control.

Check List of Equipment and Audiologic Supplies*

(1) *Hearing Evaluation Unit*

   a. Master control panel switches, meter, etc.
   b. Pure tone audiometers
   c. Masking unit
   d. Tape recorder-reproducer
   e. Disc record player
   f. Power amplifier
   g. Headphones, cushions, and headbands
   h. Loudspeaker in infinite or bass reflex baffle
   i. Disc and tape recordings of test material
   j. Talk-back unit including microphone, amplifier, headphones and monitor loud-speaker
   k. Tuning forks
   l. Microphone for live voice
   m. Peep show
   n. Calibrated noise makers

(2) *Psychogalvanic Skin Resistance Unit*

   a. Direct current galvanometer
   b. Leads and electrodes
   c. Faradic inductorium

(3) *Auditory Training Unit*

   a. Reproducer unit including microphone, record player, amplifier, loud-speaker and headphone sets
   b. Special teaching disc recordings, noise makers, etc.
   c. Skulls, anatomic models, illustrations, etc.
   d. Interoffice telephone system with amplified telephone for practice

(4) *Speech*

   a. Films for practice
   b. Hand mirrors, wall mirror, tongue blades
   c. Desk type hearing aid

* Reprinted, by permission, from Heller, M. F., and Lindenberg, P.: The private practice of auditory rehabilitation. Ann. Otol., Rhin. & Laryng. 63: 130. Copyright 1954, Annals Pub. Co.

(5) *Speech (Lip) Reading*
  a. Films for practice
  b. Motion picture projector and screen
  c. Reproducer (can be the same as for auditory training)

(6) *Hearing Aid Selection*
  a. Representative hearing aids
  b. Extra batteries for fittings
  c. Universal and stock ear inserts
  d. Fixed, common baffle for mounting hearing aids during fittings

(7) *Calibration and Repair Equipment*
  a. Vacuum tube voltmeter
  b. Soldering iron, tool kit, etc.
  c. Hearing aid battery tester

(8) *Ear Insert Equipment*
  a. Impression material
  b. Dental engine, polishing stones, buffers for adjustments

(9) *Miscellaneous*
  a. Blackboard and related supplies
  b. Toys, selected for testing as well as entertaining children

4

THE PATIENT'S HISTORY

Usually when a patient presents himself to an otologist because of impaired hearing he does so with some uneasiness. He has been experiencing, over some length of time, anxiety about himself. Is he really hard of hearing; has his attitude towards his fellows changed, or their attitude towards him? He has been embarrassed and has embarrassed others by failing to hear, or failing to hear correctly.

For example, two people are about to go their separate ways. They make their adieus when suddenly one says something to the other, who is hard of hearing. The latter turns and walks away. The speaker feels rebuffed although his companion is unaware of the incident, and their relationship has suffered a blow. It needs little imagination to realize how such incidents alter social, business, professional and economic relationships.

The man whose hearing is impaired is fearful of his job security. The woman may have similar fears, either of a threat to a job or to her domestic or social situations. The student has difficulties in his scholastic life and anticipates greater problems as he approaches a career. The young lady may have already experienced social difficulties, and fears that she is afflicted with a handicap which is a threat to marriage and a home. The mother is apprehensive about the hearing of her child; and the child with poor hearing may have grown fearful, suspicious or resentful because of the hurts he has suffered without understanding that his defective hearing, of which he knows nothing, has victimized him.

Many hard of hearing people postpone facing the reality of their hearing loss. When at last they admit the necessity of seeking help, their psychological resources may be strained to the utmost.

Most people are not too reticent about their ailments. They will talk about their operations, illnesses, ophthalmological or dermatological problems. But rarely will an individual divulge his acoustic handicap. The one expression used so frequently by hard of hearing people is, "I'm embarrassed."

But deafness is more than embarrassing; it is isolating. The normal hearing public finds difficulty in trying to communicate with the hard of hearing, and tends to shy away. The hard of hearing are hurt and afraid to expose their defect and themselves, so that two factors contribute to separate this handicapped group from society.

Parental impaired hearing contaminates a home. The acoustically handicapped mother becomes apprehensive because she fears she will be unable to hear her baby when he cries or calls. The baby who cannot attract his mother's attention may develop behavioral problems because of this seeming rejection. As tots, such children cannot understand why father or mother fails to answer or why the response is irrelevant; it even happens that a child is accused by the hard of hearing parent of having said something "wrong," when in reality the parent has failed to hear correctly. In addition, since with hearing losses defective speech patterns develop as a complication, children in homes in which one parent has defective speech may themselves learn to speak defectively.

Furthermore, patients with conductive deafness frequently reduce voice volume. Employers and associates complain that such a person mumbles, speaks too softly, makes a poor impression on the public because the speech is monotonous, dull, and difficult to hear, suggesting that the speaker is disinterested. In the home, a parent with such speech may not be heard even by the normal-hearing children, or may be misunderstood. The parent, in turn, may be angered by his child's apparent indifference.

Binaural loss of hearing is a tremendous social, educational, economic and psychological handicap. Many people can make effective use of a hearing aid, some cannot. Some patients find the aid serviceable under ideal listening conditions, but much less so under the many varied conditions of living. A short order cook in a noisy kitchen complains that although he hears well enough with the aid at home he cannot hear efficiently at work. Many people such as order clerks and dispatchers conduct their business over the telephone. Severely defective ears may be unable to hear or to understand conversation over this system.

The list of examples is inexhaustible. Some of these problems may be alleviated with relatively little effort, some are almost insurmountable.

Monaural deafness, too, causes much distress. The individual with monaural deafness cannot stroll down the street with a person on each side of him and be able to hear both companions. At round table discussions he misses the conversation on the side of his impaired ear, or he constantly gyrates to catch all the conversation coming from his impaired side. When such conferences become animated the monaurally deafened person lags behind and loses the trend of the conversation.

The person with monaural deafness usually demonstrates astereophonia. He is unable to localize the source of a sound.

If he is engrossed in some activity and is called, he looks all about, first to the side of his good ear, then everywhere until he sees the origin of the stimulus. Such persons have lost their acoustic depth perception, their acoustic spatial relationships. This is distressing and can endanger the patient who cannot localize a sound of warning such as an automobile horn, and may just as readily walk into the path of injury as turn away from it.

Monaural deafness is handicapping in many occupations. A taxicab driver complains that because of his left deafness he cannot hear potential passengers who hail him from the left side of the cab. An interviewer has his desk placed to conform with a general office plan, turns 90 degrees in his chair to bring his good ear into a conversation, and misses what his visitor says when he turns away. A lecturer at school hears only questions directed from one side of the room. A child in school sits with his good ear towards a wall, his poor ear towards the teacher. At such times he may fail to hear when called upon, which is misinterpreted as dullness, unruliness and inattention. He may suffer unearned punishment as a consequence.

Examples such as these are innumerable; each is an individual problem. Some can be resolved with some relief to the patient, others are more difficult of resolution, and some patients may not be helped at all.

Obtaining the History

For the otologist's understanding of the problems of his patient and his auditory handicap, the patient is the best textbook. Our patients teach us, if we are but willing to listen, think and learn.

Obtaining the history from a patient with a hearing im-

pairment is a little different than that of taking a history
generally. A patient with some acute pathological process
may enter the office and state that he has an acute sinusitis
or peritonsillar abscess. He has had similar experiences which
have responded to treatment. He knows what is wrong with
him this time and seeks relief. These histories are simple
and direct. But the patient with impaired hearing presents
a less simple story. His attitude toward his defect is an un-
happy one. He is resentful, bitter, angry, frightened, wor-
ried, apprehensive. Often he has come to the otologist not
of his own volition, but because of pressure from his family
or employer.

Taking a patient's history should accomplish many things.
As much as possible should be learned of the onset, origin,
course and previous treatment. We want to know how the
deafness has affected his relationships at home, at work and
at play; how it has altered his behavior; what the patient
thinks of his difficulties and what he thinks of himself;
what previous attempts have been made to alleviate his
deafness and his disappointment because of the failure of
improvement. We want to know what jobs he has lost or
failed to get, and why he has postponed seeking help for so
many years.

We inquire about his impaired hearing, how it interferes with direct conversation with only one speaker, and
with several speakers, over the phone, in noisy places, over
distances, listening to the radio and television, at church,
lectures, movies, theater, meetings. Some people hear satisfactorily in a quiet place, but under noisier conditions cannot understand the speech they hear. Some hear speech
better in the presence of noise.

We inquire further, when was the hearing loss first discovered and by whom (the patient or his associates); whether
the loss increased gradually and insidiously, or suddenly.

Have head noises or dizziness been experienced, in conjunction with the deafness, or with improvement or increased loss of hearing? Had one ear become involved before the other, are there differences between the two ears at present. Are there influences in daily living which alter the hearing or sensations in the ears: fatigue, nervousness, alcohol, tobacco, allergies, foods, drugs, atmospheric changes, flying, noises?

Is dizziness a symptom; did it precede the onset of the deafness, or appear at a later date? Has the loss of hearing increased with episodes of dizziness? Has there been nausea, vomiting, falling? Were any injuries sustained if the patient fell? If the hearing has become worse during a dizzy spell, does it recover at all when the vertiginous episode subsides?

Did the onset of deafness occur in very early life, before the age at which speech appears, or during the formative years of speech development, or after speech was fully established?

Has the patient had any medical or surgical treatment designed to improve the hearing? We also wish to know the general medical history of the patient, and if there has been any psychotherapy at any time.

Has the patient had any kind of rehabilitation? Has a hearing aid been used, was it satisfactory or if rejected why? Has he had any lip reading lessons, where, when, and by whom, and can he read lips efficiently? Similarly, the patient should be asked about speech correction lessons.

Is there a history of deafness in any member in the family, in near and distant relatives, who of these and how many relatives? What was the presumed cause of the deafness in these people?

Obtaining the history is a most significant phase in the entire investigation and in the care of the hard of hearing patient. It is a measured, steady, gentle, sympathetic approach to grasping the problem and initiating its resolution. The history sets the stage for all that will follow.

The history cannot be hurried, anticipated or taken for granted. Only by giving the patient an opportunity to talk can we learn the many ramifications of his problems. Only by permitting the patient to give of himself can he bring to the fore his fears, his anxieties, his misgivings. Only by permitting him to elaborate fully can we gain his confidence and have him sense that he has found sympathy, understanding, strength, and hope.

The technique of history taking consists basically in the willingness to listen, and when little is forthcoming in drawing the patient out of himself, out of his isolation. Obtaining a history does not consist of asking questions from a prepared questionnaire, or asking stereotyped questions. Rapport between doctor and patient enters into and predominates the discussion.

Just as life itself does not travel in a direct line as on railroad tracks, but weaves and meanders through byways as well as highways, so does the history follow these paths.

The otologist must be prepared to spend the time necessary to uncover some of what the patient has suppressed consciously and unconsciously over many years. Often a woman, and occasionally a man, will break down and weep during a gentle interview, indicating the great and suppressed anxieties. This episode can be crucial, for on it may turn the patient's willingness to accept the physician's assistance and counsel.

When a history is secured for medicolegal purposes an exact chronological sequence of events should be obtained. Was there acoustic or otic impairment prior to the injury or illness? How soon after the alleged insult were the symptoms noted? What are the characteristics and the duration of the symptoms? How have they been modified or altered subsequently? These and many other pertinent facts should be fully elucidated. A medical witness unsure of the facts may find himself on the stand in an unenviable position.

The same circumspection applies to acoustic problems alleged to be the consequence of many noisy occupations. In fairness to all concerned—the patient, the employer and his representatives, referees, judges, juries, and the doctor himself— a complete history, thorough physical examination, and exhaustive functional examinations will help to bring the facts into focus and proper perspective.

The process of getting the history encompasses even more. By the patient's recital, his allegations, by the consistency and reinforcement of the factors involved, by his contradictions, lapses, by his behavior and by his speech patterns, the otologist may be able to gauge the validity of the complaints. This, again, is of importance in medicolegal cases, since unconsciously motivated psychogenic deafness or deliberate feigning of deafness are encountered.

Some patients may present the symptom of deafness as their dominant problem when in reality they are psychologically ill. They may have auditory hallucinations, and the sounds they seem to hear may be symptomatic of their mental illness and not tinnitus at all. Other patients may have fugue-like states or momentary episodes of detachment which members of the family or friends may interpret as deafness. The otologist must be alert to many factors which in one fashion or another may simulate deafness or other otic or auditory symptoms. This is no less a problem among children.

Sometimes the crux in the history is reached after all the medical and functional studies have been completed, and possibly quite accidentally. Two experiences in clinical practice, not necessarily typical but illustrative, demonstrate the far reaches to which a history may extend. The first is that of a five year old girl who was investigated because the parents suspected that she had some impairment of hearing. The child, sweet and pretty, vehemently denied that there was anything wrong with her hearing. To her parents' astonishment and dismay she protested violently against any examination or tests. Nevertheless, she was cajoled into submitting to an examination which determined that she had a profound monaural deafness. When this was adequately determined the child was again queried when suddenly she burst into tears. After being soothed she blurted out that one of the children in the community was deaf and wore a hearing aid. All the children in the neighborhood mocked the youngster, and the little patient feared the same fate. For this reason she had tried to hide her own deafness of which she was fully aware. She was assured that she had no grounds for her fears.

The second patient was a woman of about forty years, who complained of difficulty in hearing dictation. Her employer dictated with a pipe in his mouth, which made it difficult for her to understand clearly what he said. She had noted the onset of this about three years prior to the examination. Her history seemed free of any etiologic factors. The otological examination was negative. The functional examination revealed an air conduction and bone conduction loss at 4000 cps only. The speech reception threshold by phones and in the free field were within normal limits. There was no discrimination loss. She was informed that her hearing was normal and serviceable for ordinary acoustic living. While gazing at the audiogram and almost idly speculating the otologist mused, "you know, were I forced to make just one guess at what might have caused this discrete loss, I'd say gunfire." The patient and her husband stirred with interest and the wife replied, "ten years ago for four months I had rifle and pistol practice on an indoor range." One wonders at the limitlessness of history.

The initial interview during which the history is obtained is designed also to prepare the patient psychologically for what may follow. Patients enter with the hope that they will be told their hearing loss is inconsequential, or the hope that they can find a cure in the hands of the otologist. They fear that they may be told that the loss is permanent and that it may become total, and there are no therapies to restore their hearing. Of course, some hearing defects can be alleviated by medical or surgical measures, but many hearing defects cannot.

Hence it is important for the welfare of the patient that the tenor of the interview be in such a key that the patient feels he can lower his psychological defense and feel secure in the care of the otologist. In this vein the patient may begin to become reconciled to his infirmity and to accept rehabilitation.

Evaluation of Hearing Defects in Children

The importance of the evaluation of hearing defects in infants and young children cannot be overestimated. It is during the first years of life that the brain is stimulated to grow and the personality is molded by the environment. Inability to hear normal sounds and distinguish and discriminate speech create educational and emotional deficits. Lack of hearing, lack of sensory and motor communication, inevitably penalizes intellectual and emotional maturation.

It is necessary for the infant to hear the many sounds of life as well as those of speech. During the first eighteen to twenty-four months of life, the child stores up a vocabulary and prepares to communicate his own ideas through speech. The failure of the auditory mechanism retards development in the growth of ideas and of self-expression. Since spoken and written words make concrete ideation and thinking, the failure of the auditory sensory organ, and as a corollary the failure of the development of the motor responses of speech, seriously impedes the development of the cerebral, intellectual and psychological processes.

For a clearer understanding of deafness of infancy it is desirable, when possible, to determine when the patient sustained the otic injury; prenatally, neonatally, or postnatally. Usually parents do not supect deafness in an infant until he is about nine months of age. The causative factor which produced the otic damage could have been operative at any time after conception. Accordingly, information is desired in the history with the purpose of trying to determine when the injury or defect might have been sustained.

At times there is a history of some maternal infection during the pregnancy, such as measles, pertussis, lues, influenza, or some febrile undiagnosed illness. Sometimes there is a maternal history of the ingestion of drugs, such as quinine, salicylates or alcohol. Occasionally there is a story of some physical trauma, as a blow to the abdomen of the mother. There may have been an episode of uterine bleeding during the pregnancy.

Other histories reveal prolonged strenuous labor, heavy sedation, prolonged obstetrical anesthesia. There may be a history of instrumental delivery, or breech delivery. There may have been neonatal icterus with or without evidence of Rh negativity. There may have been neonatal cyanosis, periods of apnea; the newborn may have required oxygen for some period of time.

During the first several months of life the infant may have suffered from some illness or intoxication. He may have experienced a febrile episode, often with vomiting and other symptoms. Viral infections producing precipitate perceptive deafness have been observed in the adult, and presumably will produce the same sudden damage in the infant. Infants often sustain head injuries, falling off a bed, out of a chair or carriage, or down a flight of stairs. Sometimes they are struck by falling objects. There may have been little or no evidence of significant intracranial damage, but, again, as an apparently minor head injury in the adult may produce perceptive deafness, the same kind of injury may cause deafness in the infant.

It is important for the parents to be told that the deafness is not inherited but congenital whenever this is the case; that the infant was born with deafness, or aquired it postnatally, from some extrinsic cause rather than because of some genetic defect which adversely affects the normal development of the embryonic acoustic structures. If an extrinsic cause can be determined with reasonable clinical certainty, one may be optimistic that subsequent children of this couple will be born with normal hearing.

With increasing understanding and management in the care of the new-born many hazards of the neonatal period may be reduced, thereby protecting the new-born's auditory end organ and lessening the risks of the occurrence of deafness at this level of life. The prevention of accidents and illnesses during the early months of life need not be stressed for the sake of protecting the hearing alone; it must be remembered, however, that apparently minor illnesses or accidents may have as their only sequela perceptive deafness.

In the light of this, obtaining a history from the parents may be a searching process. One wants to know why the parents suspect that the infant cannot hear; how recently this thought has been entertained. A mother may say how proud she felt because the new baby slept so soundly, undisturbed by the noises in the home. But now he still sleeps in the presence of noises which presumably should awaken him. The baby may make an effort to mimic the mother's voice, but does not respond when called by his name. He fails to turn towards her at the sound of her approach, as other children do. Occasionally he jumps because of a sudden loud sound, as if caught by surprise, but is inattentive unless the sound is unusually loud.

If the baby is at the age when speech should appear he makes no effort to speak; he may laugh or emit various vocal sounds, but no word, or rarely an occasional word, is uttered. Deaf infants will emit sounds for many months but if speech is not heard these vocal manifestations will become less and less frequent.

Additional history will be enlightening in terms of other behavioral expressions of the infant. Are his height and weight development within normal limits? Has the infant attempted to crawl, sit, stand, walk? Does he grasp at objects and play with them as do normal children of the same age. The presence of other organic or psychological pathology must be determined or excluded. The deviant behavior of some children may be interpreted as the result of deafness, but on further examination entirely different pathology may be uncovered whereas the hearing turns out to be normal. The functional examination of the pediatric patient is described in *Chapter 10.*

Chronology of Study and Care of the Hard-of-Hearing Patient*

(1) *History*
(2) *ENT Examination*

* Reprinted, by permission, from Heller, M. F., and Lindenberg, P.: The private practice of auditory rehabilitation. Ann. Otol., Rhin. & Laryng. 63: 130. Copyright 1954, Annals Pub. Co.

(3) *Tests of equilibration when indicated*

(4) *Additional medical studies when indicated*

(5) *Tests of auditory function*
   a. Pure tone threshold audiometry
      Air conduction
      Bone conduction
   b. Lateralization when indicated
   c. Stenger audiometry when indicated
   d. Recruitment audiometry when indicated
      Binaural alternate loudness balance
      Monaural loudness contours
   e. Speech reception tests
      Phones
      Free field
   f. Speech discrimination tests
      Phones
      Free field
   g. Speech to noise ratio
   h. Galvanic skin response pure tone audiometry when indicated
   i. Hearing aid selection

(6) *Impression made of auricle and meatus, model for permanent insert*

(7) *Speech analysis*

(8) *Staff consultation*

(9) *Patient consultation*
   a. Discussion of problem
   b. Recommendations
      Medical therapy
      Surgical therapy
      Rehabilitation: Hearing aid (written prescription), Auditory training, Speech (lip) reading, Speech correction, Program planning.

(10) *Follow-up services*
   a. Reexaminations and retesting
   b. Hearing aid reevaluations
   c. Studies of speech
   d. Studies of speech (lip) reading proficiency

5

PURE TONE AUDIOMETRY

The results of a test are no better than the competency of the person performing the test. Perfect equipment in the hands of someone untrained, disinterested, or unimaginatively following printed instructions will not produce consistently accurate, worth-while test results.

Testing the patient's hearing implies testing the tester's ability. Each phase of testing is based on principles. Experience and intelligence permit one to recognize when valid results are being obtained and when the results are spurious. Audiologic and otologic experience are necessary to recognize inaccuracies, inconsistencies and mistakes. Occasionally apparent paradoxes in the findings are not inconsistent.

Testing a patient's hearing is more than the investigation of some discrete defect of an organ located peripherally and physically on the lateral side of the skull. Intimately affiliated with the otic organ is a brain, a personality, a whole being, all of which are responding to test stimuli in a critical and often threatening situation. Testing a patient's hearing is really testing a whole person, and a mere pusher of buttons and twister of dials will fail utterly.

Some patients cooperate well when tested. They accept the situation with equanimity and can tolerate being scrutinized and challenged. Other patients are apathetic, tense, frightened, hostile, aggressive, resentful, indifferent, or passive. Some patients in addition to their otic physical ailment may have other physical ailments. Still other patients have an anxiety neurosis, some are obsessive compulsive, some are schizophrenic, some have other psychoses. Some patients hallucinate, some are almost catatonic; others are challenged by any test and must "pass" it. Some try to squeeze out the last bit of sound they can hear, others will stop listening once the tone drops below a loudness level which holds their interest. There is nothing routine or automatic in the testing of hearing. There are steps of procedure which follow one another, but occasionally the pattern may be changed because of the personality of the patient. It must be assumed that the otologist is expert in presenting the many tests, or enjoys the services of an audiometrician of such competency and integrity and intelligence that the latter's work can be depended upon without question.

After the history has been obtained and the otorhino-laryngological examination performed, testing of hearing is the next item on the agenda. The patient is told what he can expect and what is wanted of him. He is told that he will wear a phone or receiver over his ear through which soft sounds will be heard; when he hears a sound he is to signal that he has heard, and the sound will stop. He will then hear it a little softer and again he will signal that he has heard it and again the sound will stop. The sound will be made softer and softer until he no longer hears it.

Adults may signal in several ways. In a usual method the patient raises his hand each time he hears the sound and lowers it when the sound stops. Another signaling device permits the patient to operate a button which activates a light in view of the tester. (Some patients forget to remove the finger after having pressed the button when the tone is interrupted.)

Generally the most satisfactory signal on the patient's part is to let him respond with "yes" each time he hears the stimulus. There are several advantages to this. He participates more actively and naturally when he replies to a sound with a verbal response. He is less isolated if he is permitted to speak, which relaxes him. He may demonstrate changes in his voice volume as the tone intensity becomes greater or less, which is a good indication to the tester of the patient's subconscious reactions to the changes of loudness. This is particularly important when testing patients with deafness of non-organic origin, so-called psychogenic deafness.

Children's cooperation can be obtained by making the test a simple game. The child is given a noise-maker such as a cowbell or toy "cricket" and instructed to signal with the toy each time he hears the sound in his ear.

Air Conduction Audiometry

It is desirable to start with the intensity of each tone at about the suspected threshold of the patient's hearing. Some patients if they are first introduced to a loud sound may be unresponsive to softer ones that follow. If they learn to listen to and for soft sounds at the beginning of the test, their thresholds may be obtained more easily and rapidly. Experience has demonstrated that the 1000 cycle frequency is an effective point of departure. After the threshold of this frequency has been obtained, one may then test the ascending or descending octaves successively. The tester may prefer to start with an intensity below the patient's threshold and slowly increase the intensity until the patient signals that he has heard. The stimulus is immediately interrupted and the intensity is decreased 5 decibels and the stimulus is reintroduced. Each time the patient responds the intensity is reduced 5 decibel steps until the patient no longer indicates that he has heard.

If one ear hears normally or better than the other, the better ear should be tested first. This allows the patient to become familiar with the procedure and will also demonstrate if he is responding properly and accurately.

The poorer ear is then tested for air conduction without masking. If the air conduction thresholds between the two ears at several frequencies are no greater than 35 decibels, usually masking of the better ear is not indicated.* If the difference between the two is greater than 35 decibels at some frequencies, the better ear should be masked at those frequencies where the difference is greater. It is important to note whether there is a threshold shift of the poorer ear when the better ear is masked. Frequently the difference between the unmasked threshold and masked threshold may be only 5 decibels, which is negligible. At times the difference may be marked. The tester may find it necessary to recheck by varying the masking intensity to determine if he has masked adequately.

Masking

The purpose of masking is to eliminate temporarily the hearing of the ear which is not being tested. If the intensity of a tone stimulus entering one ear is great enough, this tone can travel through the skull, or around it, and be heard by the ear not being tested. The patient may not and usually

---

* Opinions vary among authorities. It is the author's practice to test first without masking and then with masking in order to be able to evaluate the effect of the masking. Some factors which may influence the decision are (1) lateralization and (2) the acuity of hearing of the better ear.

does not recognize that the tone is crossing over and merely reports that he hears the stimulus. One way whereby the ear not being tested can be occluded is to keep it occupied by another sound—a masking sound.

Measurements have determined that the skull has an impedance of between 55 decibels and 65 decibels. Intensities greater than 65 decibels will cross through the skull, from one side to the other, and be heard as sound by the other ear. The problem is to obtain a masking sound whose own spectrum is wide enough to embrace the frequencies of the several tones used during the test, to obtain an intensity of sound that accomplishes effective masking, and to avoid such intensities of the masking sound that would cross over to the opposite ear—the one being tested—and thereby mask both ears.

If no masking is employed, a totally deaf ear can demonstrate an apparent threshold of hearing. This is a shadow curve reflecting a response to the stimulus by the better ear. The intensity of the stimulus entering the skull on the side of the deaf ear is great enough to penetrate the skull and cross over to excite the end organ of the opposite good ear. Sufficient masking of the better ear will suppress the shadow curve. Masking of between 60 decibels and 75 decibels will usually accomplish this.

Several instruments have been used to produce a masking noise. An early masker was the Barany alarm apparatus which produced an uncalibrated rattling sound of low frequencies. The contemporary masking instruments are electric vacuum tube systems which produce either a saw tooth noise or a white noise. Many audiometers have a masking circuit built into the instrument which can be brought into play by turning on the masking switch. The intensity of the masking tone can be controlled by an attenuator.

Usually an intensity of 60 decibels of masking noise is sufficient to assure adequate masking. At times 50 decibels of masking may be sufficient, and rarely 80 decibels and more may be necessary. There does not seem to be a hard and fast rule. The tester may have to repeat the audiometry with varying intensities of masking after which he should be able to decide which test demonstrates sufficient masking, insufficient masking or over-masking. Masking is to be used discriminately, when there are appropriate indications. Routine unplanned masking may produce erroneous results just as readily as the lack of its application when masking is indicated.

An occasional patient will be met who has monaural perceptive deafness of one ear and conductive deafness of the other ear. Such a situation will tax the ingenuity of the tester but by repeated testing of each ear with and without masking of the opposite ear an accurate audiogram of each ear can be obtained.

Bone Conduction Audiometry

Bone conduction audiometry is obligatory, because the functional diagnosis is predicated on a comparison of the air conduction thresholds and the bone conduction thresholds. This is fundamental. Functional diagnosis is generally impossible unless both procedures are performed.

The technique of bone conduction audiometry is identical with that of air conduction audiometry. The bone conductor should be placed firmly against the mastoid process. Occasionally a particular point on the skull in the region of the mastoid process will be found where the tone is heard better than in the immediate vicinity. The point where the patient reports that he hears best is selected for placement of the bone conductor.

If the air conduction thresholds of both ears throughout the auditory spectrum are essentially alike, masking of either ear is usually not indicated. If the difference between the two ears is more than 35 decibels masking of the better ear may be indicated, both for air conduction and for bone conduction.

Lateralization

In an effort to determine more exactly the necessity for masking, lateralization tests for each frequency should be performed. The bone conductor is placed on the forehead in the midline. The patient is exposed to each of the frequencies of 250 cps through 4000 cps at the maximum of the attenuator. The patient reports to the tester where he hears the tone: in the head, in the midline, in the right ear or in the left ear. Some patients are not sure where they hear the tones. The patient's responses should be written on the audiogram at each frequency: *R* for lateralization to the right ear, *L* for lateralization to the left ear, and a vertical arrow if there is no lateralization. It is not unusual to find right lateralization at one frequency, left lateralization at another frequency, and no lateralization at other frequencies. Hence to report that a patient lateralizes to one ear or another without indicating the frequency and without having tested all the frequencies implies incomplete and inadequate testing for lateralization.

If lateralization is to the poorer-hearing ear (usually suggesting conductive deafness), masking of the better-hearing ear is generally unnecessary. Lateralization to the better-hearing ear invariably demands masking of this good ear when testing the poorer ear by bone conduction as well as by air conduction.

Threshold

The threshold point is not necessarily the softest tone, of least intensity, to which the patient responds at the moment. As in other physiological tests of threshold, it is an average of several repeated observations. The technique in testing hearing audiometrically is as follows: obtain, for each frequency, the last and least intensity to which the patient responds, increase intensity by 5 decibels, obtain the patient's response, decrease intensity by 5 decibels thereby bracketing the threshold point. In this way a 50 per cent recognition of the presence of the tone is obtained, and this 50 per cent average is the accepted threshold in decibels, for each specific frequency.

Caution should be exercised when exposing the tones to the patient. With long exposures, particularly at high intensities, ears may become fatigued, or adapt, thereby altering the threshold. The acuity of hearing may be reduced and erroneous thresholds will be obtained. To avoid such artifacts the tones should be exposed only briefly, particularly when the higher intensities are required. This same caution should be observed when the recruitment tests are performed (*See Chapter 6*).

Warbling and Other Devices

At about threshold some patients are not sure they are really hearing the tone. Sometimes the patient can be made more attentive by increasing the intensity just enough to remind him what he is listening for. At times warbling holds the patient's acoustic attention. Warbling consists of rapid minute changes of frequency about the frequency being tested. This minute shifting of frequency catches the patient's hearing attention as he can more readily recognize contrasting frequencies at threshold than a steady pure-tone stimulus.

A sweep frequency audiometer permits hand operation to produce warbling. The frequency selector is rotated rapidly and minutely about the frequency being tested. Some audiometers have a warbling unit built into the equipment, which when placed in the circuit automatically produces the warbling effect.

One of the problems the patient encounters is to distinguish between the tone at about threshold and his tinnitus. Warbling is one method of circumventing the interference or masking effect of the tinnitus. Another effective technique is to tell the patient to listen for the number of times he hears the tone in a quick succession of "pips." The tester will interrupt the stimulus so that the patient is exposed to it from one to four times. The patient tells the tester the number of times he has heard the tone; as long as he gives the correct numbers one can feel confident that the testing is progressing reliably. This technique is effective with some children, also, after about five years of age.

Another method is to tell the patient to hum or whistle or sing the tone when he hears it. This helps him to distinguish the tone stimulus from his tinnitus and also tends to keep him more attentive.

Occasionally a patient is loath to respond to minimum threshold stimuli. This may be psychological or may have medicolegal implications. The patient's facial expressions, fixity of the eyes and eyelids, and general body attitude offer clues by which the tester can suspect that the patient is hearing but is doubtful about having heard or is trying to conceal that he has heard.

Equipment Check

Familiarity with one's equipment is requisite for working competently and swiftly so that the patient does not tire or become confused. Familiarity with the testing techniques allows one to vary the procedure and thereby check on the patient's reactions, and to assure oneself that the replies are reasonably consistent and accurate. Some understanding of how and why the equipment works as it does helps the observer to recognize that a test may or may not be progressing satisfactorily. The equipment may develop defects. It comprises wires, vacuum tubes, attenuators, frequency selector systems, electric contacts, soldered electric connections, air conduction receivers, bone conductors, magnetic tape recorders, disc players, amplifying systems, loud speakers and many other parts. A defect in any of these can alter the calibration of the equipment. For example, electric contacts may corrode, become dusty or dirty. These will interfere with the flow of electrical impulses or may produce scratchy noises in the receivers which the patient will hear and assume are a test tone, and will reply accordingly.

It is good practice to turn on the current of the system each working day, and leave it on until the day's work is completed. Turning off the current after each patient has been tested permits the system to heat and cool unevenly, thereby altering its performance. The wear and tear of keeping the current on is negligible nor is the cost appreciable. It is advisable at least once a week to perform an audiometric test on oneself or someone else in the office, to check the operation of the equipment. Such a check is not time-consuming and it avoids the sudden discovery, just as one wishes to test a patient, that the system is not in calibration.

Air conduction receivers and bone conductors are rather

delicate instruments, manufactured to perform faithfully and with fidelity. They can be damaged by falling to the floor or by some other similar impact. Over the years their acoustical characteristic may change. If a receiver has been jarred, one should test its function before using it clinically. Audiometry should be performed on a normal hearing subject, who has been tested on previous occasions. If abnormal audiograms are obtained the receiver should be returned to the manufacturer for repair, recalibration or replacement. Since these receivers are expensive to replace, and since time is lost while a receiver is useless, they demand respect and care.

A certain feel for the equipment and the testing techniques can be obtained by testing oneself. In doing so one realizes the sensations and efforts to listen to threshold intensities. One becomes attuned to the subjectivity of tests and learns to anticipate the wonderment or bewilderment of many patients who may only partially realize the nature of these tests. When a patient is seated in a room which is sound treated, behind a closed door, and subjected to a test the outcome of which is of critical importance to him, the observer's empathy contributes to his comfort and cooperation.

The Audiogram

Uniformity of notations on the audiograms is desirable. There is growing a general agreement whereby certain symbols have been standardized (Fig. 2). One satisfactory series of symbols is as follows:

(1) *Right Ear, Air Conduction*

A circle at each frequency indicates the threshold. The

NAME OF
PATIENT _____ DATE _____

(FIRST)   (MIDDLE)   (LAST)

AUDIOGRAM

(AUDIOMETER)

AVERAGE HEARING →

HEARING LOSS (DECIBELS)

-20 -10 0 10 20 30 40 50 60 70 80 90 100

FREQUENCY: 125 250 500 1000 2000 4000 8000

LEGEND.

	RIGHT EAR (RED)	LEFT EAR (BLUE)
AIR CONDUCTION	o—o (WITH LEFT EAR MASKED) △—△	●--● (WITH RIGHT EAR MASKED) □--□
NO RESPONSE		
BONE CONDUCTION		
NO RESPONSE		

RECRUITMENT

☐ BINAURAL ALTERNATE BALANCE
☐ EQUAL LOUDNESS CONTOUR

0 10 20 30 40 50 60 70 80 90 100

FREQUENCY: 125 250 500 1000 2000 4000 8000

TINNITUS

☐ CONSTANT ☐ INTERMITTENT ☐ NONE	RIGHT EAR	LEFT EAR
CHARACTER		
FREQUENCY		
LEVEL (db)		

SUMMARY OF HEARING EVALUATION

	SPEECH RECEPTION THRESHOLD (db)	SPEECH DISCRIMINATION LOSS LEVEL (db) NOISE	PBs	% LOSS	PURE TONES AVERAGE LOSS 500-2000 (db)	% LOSS (AMA)	STENGER ☐POS. ☐NEG. INFERRED THRESHOLD 500	1000	2000	DOERFLER-STEWART	TOLERANCE LIMIT (db)
BINAURAL											
RIGHT											
LEFT											

RELIABILITY OF RESPONSES:

NOTES-

Fig. 2—Record form for hearing tests and hearing evaluation.

thresholds are connected by a solid line. When a red pencil, (red for right ear) is used, the identification is emphasized.

A triangle is used instead of a circle to indicate that left ear is masked.

(2) *Left Ear, Air Conduction*

A dot or "X" at each frequency indicates the threshold. The thresholds are connected by a broken line. A blue pencil may be used for contrast.

A square is used instead of a dot or "X" to indicate that right ear is masked.

(3) *Right Ear, Bone Conduction*

A box is drawn open to the right, and placed to the left of the frequency ordinate, with red pencil.

(4) *Left Ear, Bone Conduction*

A box is drawn open to the left, and placed to the right of the frequency ordinate, with blue pencil.

(5) *No Response*

When a patient fails to hear a tone at the maximum output of the audiometer the appropriate symbol *with an arrow head or dart added* is inscribed on the audiogram at the junction of the frequency ordinate and its maximum intensity abscissa. This indicates that the patient has been tested and has failed to hear at such frequencies either by bone conduction or air conduction or both.

The shape and structure of these symbols permit them to be grouped neatly together when all the thresholds at a frequency fall at the same point. There is no advantage to linking the bone conduction threshold symbols by lines.

Familiarity with a uniform system of signs permits ready interpretation. The elimination of additional and unnecessary characters and lines makes for neatness and legibility. The appropriate symbols should be recorded on the audiogram, indicating that air conduction and bone conduction testing has been performed at each frequency. There will be no misunderstanding as to whether or not all the frequencies have been tested, and what responses the patient has demonstrated.

Functional Diagnosis

The distinguishing feature contained in audiograms is the relationship between the air conduction thresholds and the bone conduction thresholds. An audiogram which portrays only air conduction thresholds depicts the threshold of hearing for pure tones. It depicts the combined function of both the tympanic structures and the neural elements. But with air conduction thresholds alone, one cannot know audiometrically whether the lesion responsible for the hearing loss involves the middle ear conducting apparatus or the sensory end organ and neural tracts. When bone conduction thresholds are plotted, also, a differential may be demonstrable. An observer cannot determine from the configuration of an audiogram the kind of pathology which has caused the deafness. The pathological diagnosis is based on sound medical investigation only.

Perceptive Deafness

When raised air conduction thresholds and bone conduction thresholds are practically identical a functional diagnosis of perceptive, nerve, deafness is tenable (Figs. 3, 4, 5).

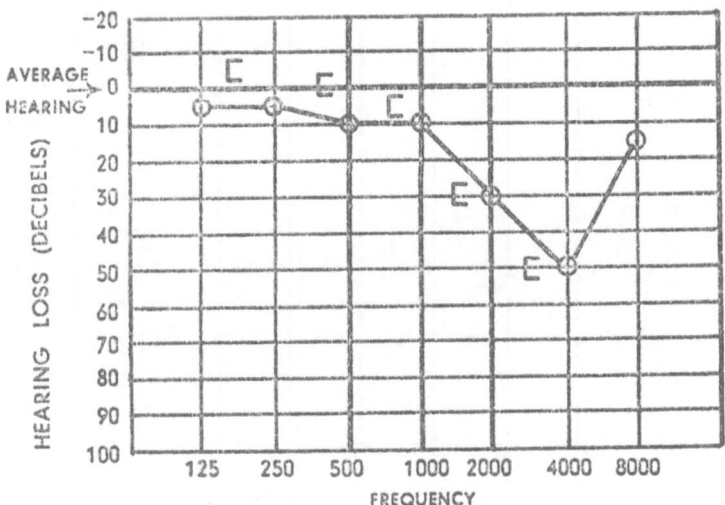

Fig. 3—Pure tone audiogram: right perceptive deafness, mild.

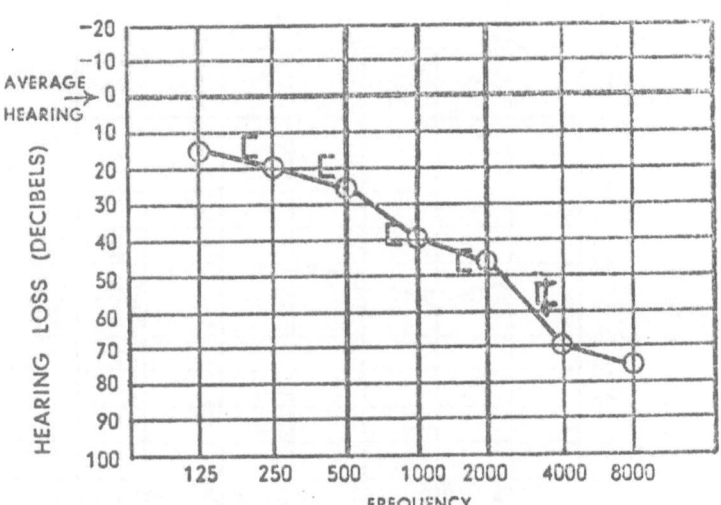

Fig. 4—Pure tone audiogram: right perceptive deafness, moderate, no bone conduction at 4000 cps.

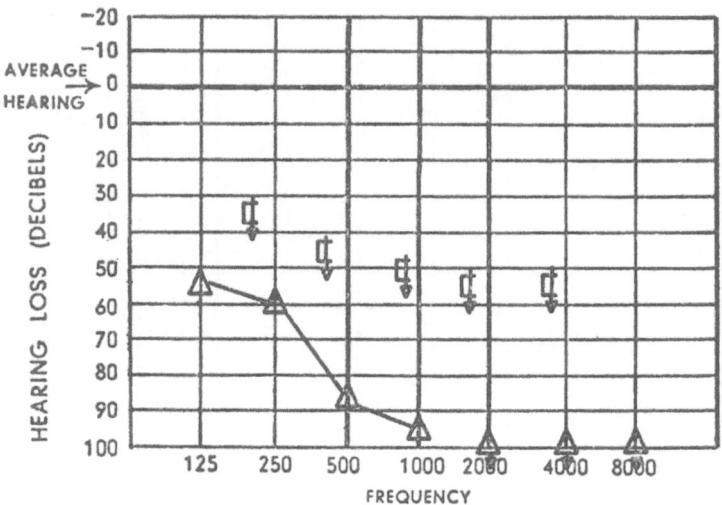

Fig. 5—Pure tone audiogram: right perceptive deafness, severe, left normal hearing ear masked both for air conduction and for bone conduction.

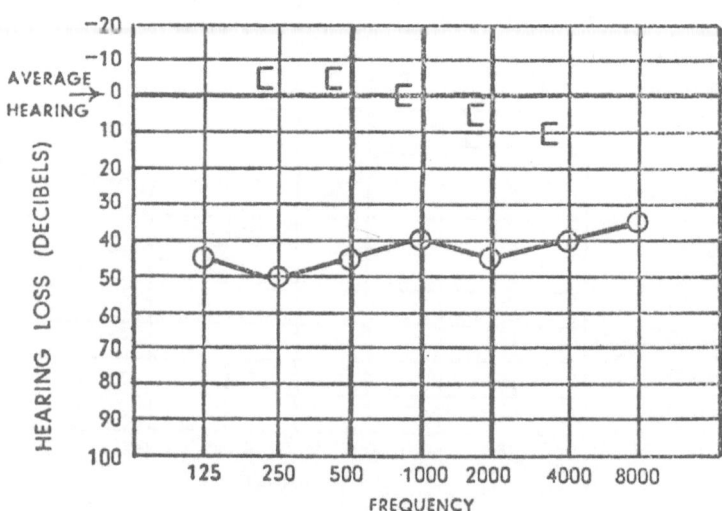

Fig. 6—Pure tone audiogram: right conductive deafness.

Conductive Deafness

When the bone conduction thresholds are approximately normal and the air conduction thresholds are raised (poor) the functional diagnosis is that of conductive deafness (Fig. 6).

Mixed Deafness

Some audiograms reflect a functional loss suggesting a mixed, or combined, deafness. There is middle ear, conductive, deafness and also perceptive deafness (Fig. 7).

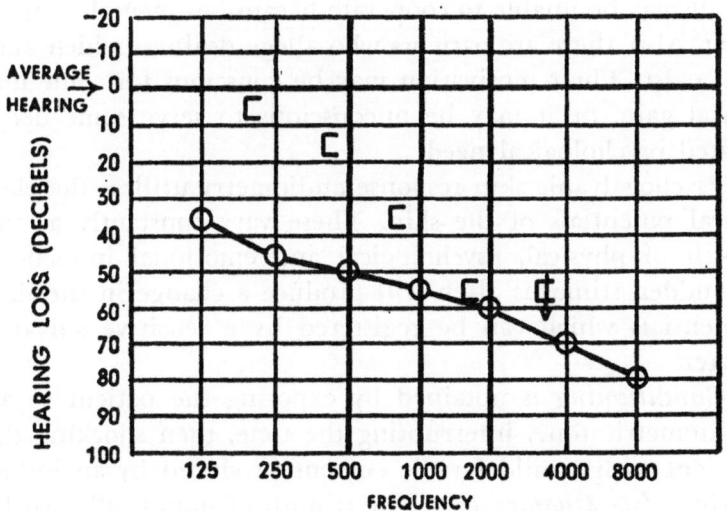

Fig. 7—Pure tone audiogram: right mixed deafness.

Psychogalvanic Skin Response Audiometry

Psychogalvanic skin response audiometry is a method of testing hearing with an audiometer by means of a conditioning process different from that ordinarily used. In routine audiometric testing the patient is instructed to signal each time he hears the test sound. These responses of the patient to an arbitrary acoustic stimulus are essentially artificial but purposeful as a means whereby the patient knows that the tester becomes aware the patient has heard the tone. Each time the patient signals he indicates that he has heard. Psychologically the test situation has become a conditioning experiment.

There are times when this kind of conditioning cannot be effectively obtained. Infants and very young children obviously cannot produce a predetermined motor response to communicate their awareness of test tones. Occasionally an adult may be unable to cooperate because of mental retardation. Also, there are patients who allege deafness which does not exist. Their motivation may be conscious for some material gain, or it may be unconscious to serve some deep-seated psychological need.

Psychogalvanic skin response audiometry utilizes the electrical potentials of the skin. These vary constantly as the result of physical, psychological and emotional influences. A sudden stimulus often will produce a change in the skin potentials which can be registered by a sensitive galvanometer.

Conditioning is obtained by exposing the patient to an audiometric tone, interrupting the tone, then shocking the patient with a mild faradic current produced by an inductorium (*see Chapter 13*). The stimuli of sound followed by a mild shock are repeated until conditioning has been established. The patient, at some deeper than conscious level, will equate the innocuous stimulus of sound with the unpleasant stimulus of electric shock, to which stimulus he will react.

After conditioning has been established, the shock stimulus is no longer employed. When the tone is heard—as long as the conditioning remains effective—the patient responds with momentary variations in his skin potentials. These brief changes are registered by the galvanometer and can be observed. With experience in this procedure the tester recognizes which changes in skin potentials are secondary to the stimulation produced by the test sound.

The duration of conditioning varies considerably. Occasionally the conditioning deteriorates as the audiometric testing is being performed, and when this occurs reconditioning with the shock will have to be repeated. In some patients the original conditioning may be maintained throughout the entire testing operation for all the frequencies. Frequently the patient must be conditioned when each new frequency is explored.

The procedure is as follows: A frequency is selected—1000 cps is a convenient point of departure—at an intensity which the tester thinks the patient can hear. The sequence of stimulation to effect conditioning is tone, interrupt, shock, interrupt, pause; tone, interrupt, shock, interrupt, pause; this sequence is repeated several times. There is evidence that the conditioning has been established when the galvanometer indicates the patient's response to the sound before the shock occurs. Pure tone audiometry is performed while the tester notes the behavior of the galvanometer with each stimulation of the tone. When the galvanometer no longer indicates a response, the threshold of hearing is considered to be the last decibel value at which the galvanometer responded.

Results are not uniformly satisfactory. As in so many tests, valid conclusions sometimes can be made, at other times the evidence is inconclusive.

Some factors which have nullified successful psychogalvanic skin response audiometric testing are: (a) Inadequate conditions where the patient's skin is so dry that even if an electrolyte is used at the contact of the skin and electrodes of the galvanometer no responses are observed; (b) Insulation, when the skin of the fingers and hands is thickly cornified; (c) Movement; some patients are so active that they keep the galvanometer in constant agitation, so that meter movements induced by sound stimulus cannot be distinguished from adventitious bodily movements.

Peep Show

Audiometry with a peep show involves a conditioning process a little different from the ordinary hand signaling. The purpose of using a peep show is to entertain the child and to reward him when he signals that he has heard. As described in the chapter on equipment, the tester has a double interrupter switch interposed between the audiometer peep show and the patient. When the tester turns his switch to "on" the tone signal arrives at the receiver or loud speaker and the peep show electric switch is "armed." If the patient pushes his switch the interior of the peep show cabinet will be illuminated and the toys can be seen rotating on the turn table. When the tester turns his interrupter switch to "off" the tone is interrupted and the light in the cabinet is extinguished. The child must wait until he again hears a sound before he can successfully light up the cabinet and see the toys. When the child becomes conditioned to this situation, pure tone threshold audiometry throughout the auditory spectrum for each ear is performed, during which the patient signals each time he hears the tone by operating his switch and causing the cabinet to be illuminated.

6_____

RECRUITMENT

Recruitment of loudness is an acoustic phenomenon observed in some cases of perceptive deafness. Not all ears with perceptive deafness recruit, but recruitment signifies perceptive deafness. Recruitment in hearing indicates that the locus of the pathology causing the perceptive deafness is probably in the cochlear structures. Normal-hearing ears do not demonstrate recruitment, nor do ears with conductive deafness. In all probability recruitment does not occur in perceptive deafness due to retrocochlear lesions, although final opinion on this must be held in abeyance.

Recruitment is the response of an ear with impaired hearing to a sound stimulus of an intensity above its threshold of hearing, enabling the ear to hear the sound as loud as if the hearing of this ear were not impaired. An ear which recruits demonstrates subnormal sensitivity at low intensities but at higher intensities appears to approach normal sensitivity. You may recall that Grandma complained you were mumbling, but that when you talked loud enough for her to hear you she complained you were shouting. Quite right. You were shouting and she was recruiting and your voice was as loud to her as it sounded to you.

Some impaired ears behave differently from other impaired ears at threshold intensities and at above threshold intensities. This has diagnostic significance. Recruitment tests may substantiate the diagnosis of conductive deafness. The tests may substantiate the diagnosis of nerve deafness due to cochlear pathology. They may also suggest as cause of the deafness the presence of pathology more centrally situated within the cranium. The clinical application of the phenomenon of recruitment described by Fowler opened up a new approach to understanding of cochlear physiology and functional pathology. Since his original clinical observations of binaural alternate loudness balance, considerable research has been performed for the further investigation of this fascinating subject, and undoubtedly much more knowledge of the behavior of the cochlea will be developed based on studies of recruitment. Shortly after Fowler's publications, Reger described the clinical application of interfrequency matching, which generally is expressed as "monaural loudness contours."

In a patient who has one normal hearing ear and one ear with perceptive deafness due to cochlear pathology, recruitment can readily be demonstrated by the technique of binaural alternate-loudness balance. If there is deafness of both ears they cannot be used for comparative exploration, and each ear must be matched against itself. One test for this is monaural loudness contours.

Binaural Alternate-Loudness Balance

Complete Recruitment

Let us assume that the right ear has a normal threshold for hearing throughout the auditory spectrum, and that the left ear demonstrates a flat loss of 50 decibels both for air conduction and bone conduction. Although an audiometer with one receiver can be used, the test is more easily performed with a two-channel audiometer with two air conduction receivers. Place a receiver over each ear.* Set the frequency selector for example at 1000 cps. Set each attenuator at 10 decibels above the threshold of each respective ear. Stimulate one ear, interrupt, stimulate the other ear, interrupt. The patient has been instructed to report in which ear the tone sounds louder. Let us assume he says the sound is louder in his poor left ear. We increase the intensity in the right ear and repeat the maneuver of matching the two ears. We continue to increase the intensity until ultimately he reports the loudness in the two ears as equal; possibly 45 decibels in the right ear and 60 decibels in the left ear. Then we raise the intensity in the left ear to 70 decibels and by comparing the ears, as before, we now find that 60 decibels in the right ear and 70 decibels in the left ear seem equally loud. Again, we add another 10 decibels to the left ear up to 80 decibels and compare. We now observe that 80 decibels in both ears sound equally loud to the patient. We had to add 80 decibels to the right ear and only 30 decibels to the left ear, above their respective thresholds, for the tone to sound equally loud at the same intensity at the same frequency. At 80 decibels the left ear caught up to the normal right ear. The left ear demonstrates recruitment (Fig. 8).

Over-recruitment

Let us go one step further. We now stimulate the right ear with an intensity of 90 decibels and find that only 85 decibels are needed in the left ear to sound as loud as 90 decibels in the normal-hearing right ear. The left ear has over-recruited. The left ear is oversensitive. This over-

---

* If a single channel audiometer is used, the patient holds the receiver to one ear and listens to the stimulus. On command of the tester the patient transfers the receiver to the other ear and listens to the stimulus. The receiver is transferred from ear to ear as binaural matching is performed.

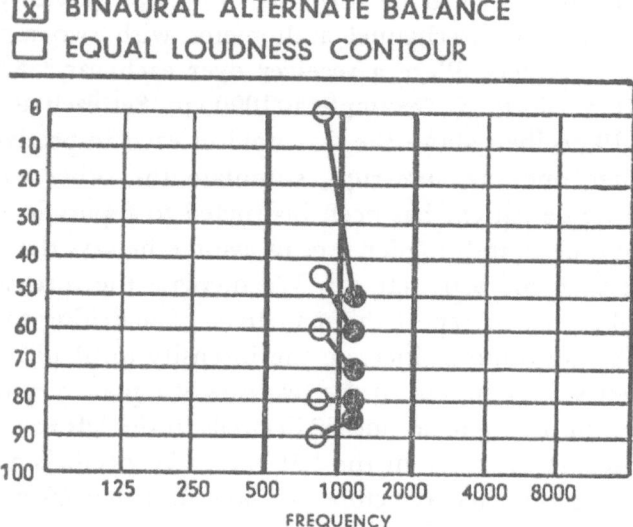

Fig. 8—Binaural alternate-loudness balance at 1000 cps: left deafness, complete recruitment at 80 db, over-recruitment at 90 db.

recruitment is additional evidence of abnormal function of the cochlear mechanism. Over-recruitment is not necessarily demonstrable when an ear recruits.

Having performed the test of binaural alternate-loudness balance at one frequency, we can proceed to study the other frequencies similarly. As we obtain this information we plot it on an audiometric form, as part of the permanent record.

Conductive Deafness, Absence of Recruitment

Now we shall assume another example of monaural deafness. The right ear has a normal threshold of 0 decibels throughout the spectrum, and again the left ear has a flat loss of 50 decibels. The bone conduction of the left ear is normal. We follow the same steps for balancing the two ears and, no matter how much we increase the intensity in the left ear, the matching continues to demonstrate a difference of about 50 decibels, within the limits of the audiometer. Even when we stimulate the left ear with an intensity of 100 decibels, the loudness which the patient experiences is only equal to the loudness which the patient experiences in the right ear at 50 decibels (Fig. 9). The left ear lags consistently behind the right ear by a measured difference of approximately 50 decibels, it does not "catch up" with the right ear, it does not recruit. We therefore conclude that the impedence of the middle ear, due to whatever pathology we had previously noted during the otological physical examination, persists regardless of the intensity with which the ear is stimulated.

Perceptive Deafness, Absence of Recruitment

A third example can be offered. The air conduction thresholds of the ears are as described in the two previous instances. However, as in the first example, the bone conduction threshold of the left ear is 50 decibels, the same as the air conduction threshold. The ears are matched, but this time the observations are similar to those in the second example, the patient with left conductive deafness. Recruitment cannot be demonstrated in this third patient with left perceptive deafness. As previously stated, it is the current thinking that recruitment is a function of the cochlear system and that the observation of perceptive deafness without recruitment implies that a retrocochlear lesion is responsible. Since expanding lesions and vascular lesion in the posterior cranial fossa, among others, may cause deafness, the diagnostic implications of perceptive deafness without recruitment are evident.

Incomplete Recruitment

In a final example of recruitment in monaural deafness,

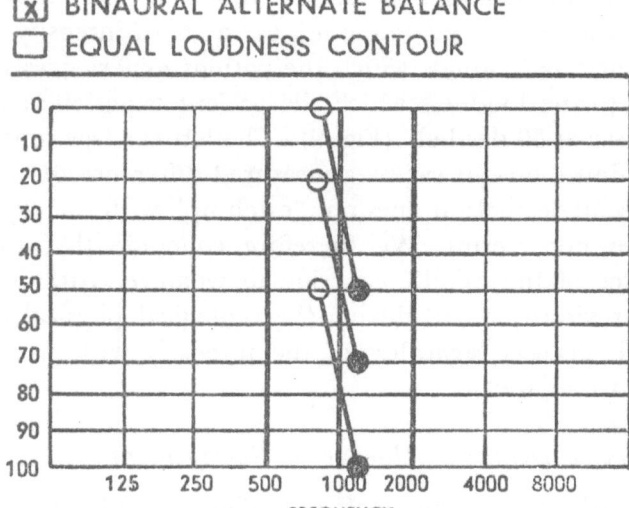

Fig. 9—Binaural alternate-loudness balance at 1000 cps: left deafness, no recruitment.

the right ear demonstrates normal hearing and the left ear demonstrates mixed deafness. The loss of hearing for the left ear by air conduction is greater than the bone conduction loss but the latter threshold is not normal. Binaural alternate-loudness balancing reveals that the left ear tends to recruit but that the recruitment is incomplete. Since this ear has both impedence (middle ear) deafness and neural (cochlear) deafness, there will be evidence of the cochlear loss by the partial recruitment and also evidence of the middle ear pathology by the partial lack of recruitment (Fig. 10).

Demonstration

As an interlude let us perform an experiment. After determining the threshold of two normally hearing ears in one subject, we pack one external auditory meatus with cotton

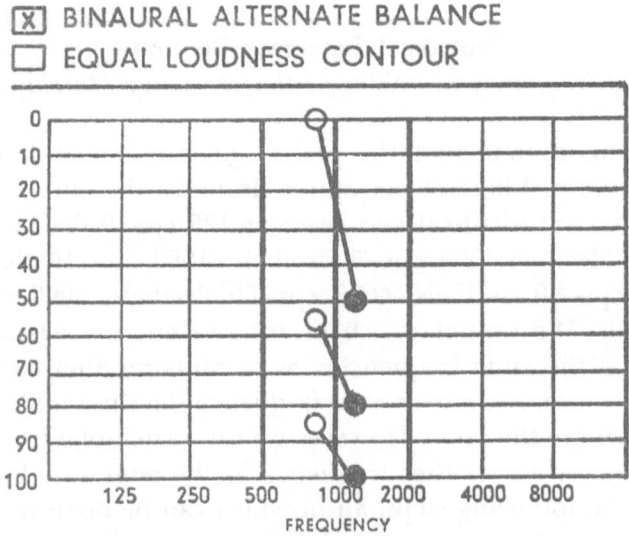

Fig. 10—Binaural alternate-loudness balance at 1000 cps: left deafness, incomplete recruitment.

saturated with some bland oil or ointment. We then perform routine air conduction audiometry to determine the hearing loss produced by the packing. We will find that the occluded ear demonstrates a raised (poor) threshold for air conduction, and temporarily demonstrates conductive deafness.

We now perform the test of binaural alternate-loudness balance. As previously described, the conductively deaf ear will be matched and balanced against the normal opposite ear at each frequency. We learn that we cannot find a common intensity where the tone will sound equally loud to both ears. The "poor" ear cannot catch up to the good ear; it will always lag behind. The intensity difference between the two ears remains approximately the same as the original difference of their thresholds. We have demonstrated that conductive deafness does not recruit (Fig. 9).

Monaural Loudness Contours
Bifrequency Matching; Interfrequency Matching

Let us assume that the patient presents an audiometric threshold of bilateral perceptive deafness; the curves of the two ears are identical and read: at 125 cps—0 decibels, 250 cps—5 decibels, 500 cps—5 decibels, 1000 cps—10 decibels, 2000 cps—40 decibels, 4000 cps—50 decibels, 8000 cps—60 decibels. We cannot match or balance one ear against the other at the same frequencies, as in binaural alternate-loudness balance, because at each frequency the thresholds of the two ears are the same. However we can match one frequency in an ear with another frequency in the *same* ear. We perform the following steps, all of which can be done with one audiometer but are accomplished more rapidly with a two-channel system:

The air conduction receiver is placed over one ear. The frequency selector is set at a frequency where the patient demonstrates a loss, as at 2000 cps. The attenuator is set at 10 decibels above the threshold, which in this example would be 50 decibels. The second frequency selector is set at a lower frequency—at 1000 cps. The attenuator is set at 10 decibels above this threshold, which would be 20 decibels. The tones will be introduced into one receiver successively with the result that the ear being tested will hear 1000 cps at 20 decibels and momentarily later 2000 cps at 50 decibels (stimulate at 1000 cps with 20 decibels, interrupt, stimulate at 2000 cps with 50 decibels, interrupt). The patient reports whether the first tone or the second tone seemed louder to him. Assume that he states that the second tone (2000 cps) sounded louder. Leave the attenuator setting of 2000 cps at 50 decibels and increase the intensity of 1000 cps, let us say, to 40 decibels. Stimulate at 2000 cps with 50 decibels, in-

☒ EQUAL LOUDNESS CONTOUR

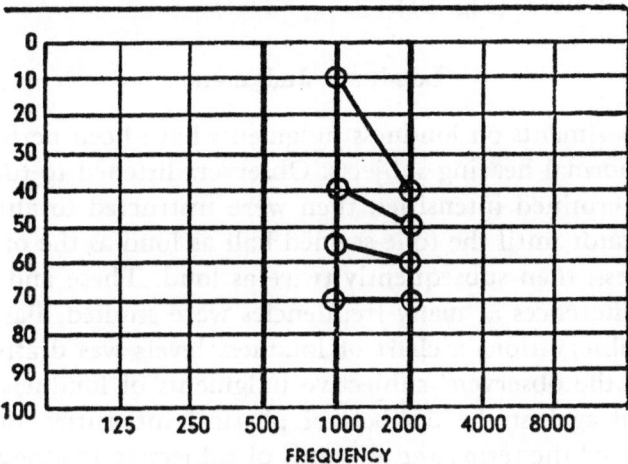

Fig. 11—Monaural (equal) loudness contours: right deafness at 2000
cps, complete recruitment at 70 decibels.

terrupt, stimulate at 1000 cps with 40 decibels, interrupt.
The patient now reports the second tone (1000 cps) sounds
as loud to him as the first tone (2000 cps). Next increase
the intensity of 2000 cps to 60 decibels and leave the attenuator of 1000 cps at 40 decibels. Stimulate at 1000 cps, interrupt, stimulate at 2000 cps, interrupt. The patient states
that 2000 cps sounds louder. Increase the intensity of 1000
cps until it sounds as loud to the patient as 2000 cps. This
time we find that 1000 cps at 55 decibels sounds as loud to
this ear as 2000 cps at 60 decibels. We will now set the 2000
cps selector at 70 decibels and upon exploration we learn
that 1000 cps at 70 decibels sounds as loud to the patient as
2000 cps at 70 decibels. The two intensities seem equally
loud to the same ear although the thresholds of hearing for
this ear at the two frequencies differ by 30 decibels. Although
there was a raised (poorer) threshold at 2000 cps, when the
intensity was increased sufficiently the ear heard this tone

as loud as it heard another tone—1000 cps—which had a normal threshold (Fig. 11).

Loudness Judgment

Experiments on loudness judgments have been performed with normal hearing subjects. Observers listened to tones of predetermined intensities, then were instructed to alter the attenuator until the tone seemed half as loud as the original loudness, then subsequently twice as loud. These and other size differences at many frequencies were studied. Based on such observations a chart of loudness levels was drafted, in which the observers' subjective judgments of loudness were plotted against the decibels of physical intensities. Stevens employed the term *sone* as a unit of subjective loudness; one sone is the loudness to a normal hearing ear of 40 decibels of intensity of a 1000 cps tone.

It was observed that, with the same decibel increments, the loudness for low frequencies grows more rapidly than for high frequencies. Hence when monaural recruitment is observed by interfrequency matching of a low frequency and a high frequency, although the intensities, in decibels, are the same and the apparent loudness of the two frequencies may appear to be the same, this may not necessarily be a 1:1 matching. Since, clinically, our purpose is to learn whether recruitment is present in a given instance, the quantitative values may be of relative consideration.

The question may be raised at times which test should be performed, binaural alternate-loudness balance or monaural loudness contours. It may be possible to perform both tests on a single patient. One ear may have a normal threshold while the other ear demonstrates unequal losses, the thresholds being at different levels. Both tests can be performed in such an instance (Figs. 12 and 13). Some patients may

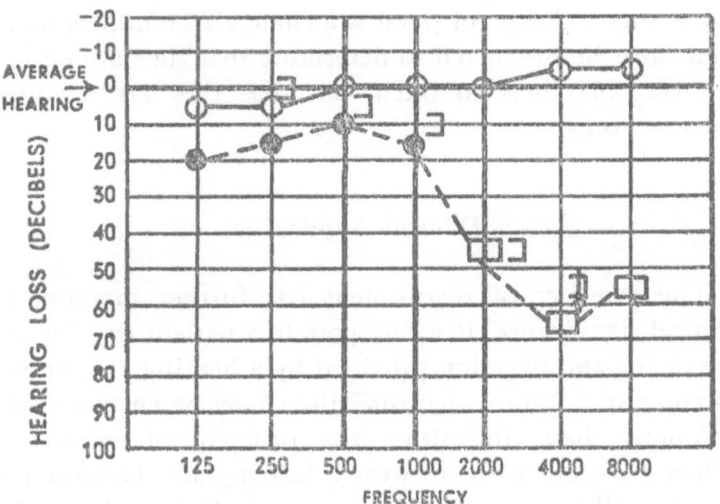

Fig. 12—Pure tone audiogram: left perceptive deafness. See Fig. 13 for recruitment tests.

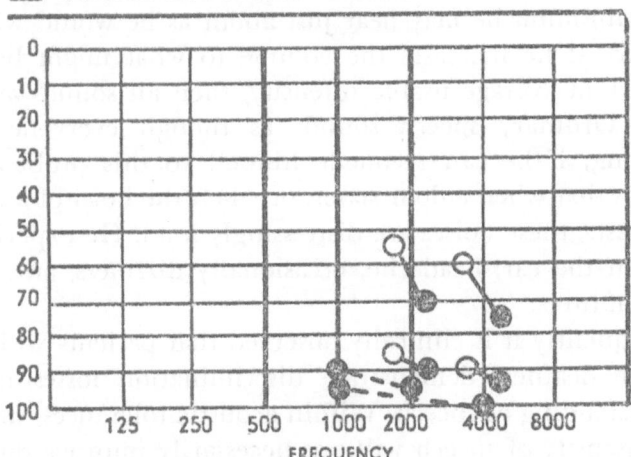

Fig. 13—Binaural alternate-loudness balance and monaural (equal) loudness contours demonstrated by one ear: left perceptive deafness. See Fig. 12 for audiogram.

think that a change of pitch is a change in loudness, so that they must be instructed to determine that they are deciding not on differences in pitch, but that they are measuring loudness only.

Clinical Application

The presence of recruitment has further practical and clinical significance. If we propose to a patient that he make use of the amplification provided by a hearing aid, we want to know in advance what difficulties may be encountered.

Among these difficulties is a problem of recruitment. When a patient plans to wear a hearing aid, he anticipates that he will hear as a normal-hearing individual hears. This is what he wants. But if he requires amplification of such a magnitude that the ordinary sounds he hears through the aid are abnormally loud, he will rebel against the use of the aid. He notices that if he turns the volume of the aid down to a minimum he may hear just about as he would without the aid. If he increases the volume to what might be considered an average usable intensity, then all sounds are too loud. Ordinary speech sounds as though everyone were shouting; if he can reconcile himself to this problem, he notices that when a door slams, or when the horn of a motor car blasts, these noises are distressingly loud. He experiences pain in the ear, headache, occasionally dizziness, and other discomfitures.

Frequently it is clinically observed that patients with perceptive deafness demonstrate discrimination losses in the understanding of speech. Within acoustic tolerances, increasing intensity of speech will not necessarily improve discrimination. Often a level of intensity is reached at which the patient's discrimination reaches its maximum, less than 100 per cent, after which further increases in intensity cause an increasing loss of discrimination.

Discrimination losses are observed in perceptive deafness, usually among patients who recruit. Accordingly when recruitment is found by the tests for it, discrimination losses can be anticipated. When prescribing a hearing aid, the otologist must anticipate that raising the volume of speech to which the patient listens may not improve the hearing for discrimination and may even aggravate the discrimination difficulties.

Hence the study of recruitment has diagnostic significance, prognostic implications, and research possibilities. In the functional examination of hearing, recruitment tests should be included whenever possible.

Subjective Factors

Recognition must be given to the mechanism beyond the ear; to the brain which is participating in these tests as well as the patient's psychological structure. Because still other factors may be involved, a further consideration must be entertained.

In performing the binaural alternate-loudness balance test, if one ear—for example, the right—is stimulated first each time, the patient may give consistent responses and appear to be able to make a valid comparison between the two ears. Whether or not recruitment is elicited is immaterial at this moment. We observe that the patient seems sure of his own observations. However, if we vary the procedure so that at one step in the matching the right ear is stimulated first and then the left, and at the next step the left ear first and then the right, we may note that the patient's responses are not as consistent as they first appeared to be. These variations may be physiological, functional, or psychological. It is well, therefore, to vary the order of testing arbitrarily until there is assurance that—regardless of which ear is first stimulated—consistencies in responses can or cannot be determined.

This applies also to the monaural loudness contour test, in beginning either with the lower frequency or the higher frequency and subsequently varying the order. Again a greater validity can be established.

Difference Limen

We now turn to the problem of determining the presence or absence of recruitment in those ears whose audiometric thresholds do not lend themselves to the technique of binaural alternate-loudness balance or of monaural loudness contours.

When we perform routine clinical audiometry we accept as the threshold of hearing a 50 per cent response at a frequency with a certain intensity. Some patients, particularly those with perceptive deafness, respond 100 per cent of the time at one intensity and fail to respond 100 per cent of the time at an intensity of 5 decibels less. Their 50 per cent response threshold must be somewhere between the two intensities. Let us assume that a patient's 50 per cent response is between 50 and 45 decibels. With an attenuator of 5 decibel gradations we cannot obtain a 50 per cent response, we know only that it is less than 50 and more than 45 decibels.

With a more discrete attenuator we can expose the patient to very small increases in intensity. The smaller the difference in intensity that an ear can detect in subjective terms as a change of loudness, the more sensitive that ear may be than another ear which requires greater increases in intensity before it recognizes an increase in loudness. Accordingly, an ear which can detect small increases in intensity as increases in loudness may be recruiting, and the ear which requires larger increases in intensity may not be recruiting.

Several clinical audiometers have been designed with an amplitude modulator, whereby the intensity can be increased in steps of fractions of a decibel. The pulsing rate can be modified from 2 to 12 pulses per second, depending upon the specifications of the manufacturer. Two to 4 pulsations per second seems to be a satisfactory rate for clinical testing.

After the threshold of a frequency has been determined, the *difference limen*, D. L., can be sought by noting how much more intensity in fractions of a decibel is needed before the patient, or subject, notices some change in the tone.

D. L. is the smallest change in a given property of sound necessary to produce an observable change in sensation. The D. L. may be normal, abnormally small, or abnormally large. An abnormally small D. L. may indicate an increased sensitivity of the ear, and an abnormally large D. L. may imply decreased sensitivity of the ear.

Hirsh, in a recent study of a group of patients, has compared their D. L.'s with the recruiting evidence as obtained by binaural or interfrequency matching, depending on each particular audiometric configuration. It was concluded that a correlation could not be established, and that there is insufficient clinical experience and evidence to warrant the acceptance of the D. L. as a measurement of recruitment. Considerably more investigation is desirable before the D. L. can be accepted as a valid estimate of recruitment, comparing favorably with the two established tests.

Difference Limen Difference

Of the several techniques which have been developed to elicit the D. L., only the difference limen difference (D. L. D.) test will be described. The patient is informed that he will hear the tone continuously, but that he will eventually observe that the steady tone will appear as a beat. He is to report when he becomes aware of the beat.

A frequency, usually 1000 cps first, is selected on the audiometer at 10 decibels above the threshold of the frequency and exposed to the patient through the air conduction receiver. The amplitude modulator is set in operation. At some point the patient reports that a beat of the tone is recognized. The decibel values are noted and the test is repeated until, after several trials, an average can be estimated. The attenuator is then raised to 40 decibels above the threshold, and the procedure is repeated at this higher level. The average decibel value of several trials is again obtained. The difference between the decibel increment obtained at 10 decibels above threshold and at 40 decibels above threshold is the D. L. D. Smaller differences in increments in decibels presumably indicate an increased sensitivity, and also presumably this is evidence of recruitment. Greater differences in increments in decibels presumably indicate a lesser sensitivity of the ear and an absence of recruitment. The several frequencies of the spectrum can be studied in this dual manner and the differences recorded. Jerger's original paper contains a description of his method of charting the results, whereby the D. L. D. is estimated.

7

DEAFNESS OF NONORGANIC ORIGIN

Hearing ultimately is a psychological experience. Certain physical environmental changes act as stimuli which alter the minute-by-minute status of the organic physiological receptor acoustic apparatus. The stimulus must be of such dimensions that changes will occur in the receptors. This receptor system is part of a hierarchy in which the psychological mechanism plays a dominant role.

One category of problems with which the otologist is confronted has to do with patients whose receptor systems are impaired, so that an amount of defective hearing results. Another category concerns patients whose receptors function satisfactorily but whose psychological interpretation of acoustic stimuli becomes distorted, perverted, or is rejected. When tests are utilized in identifying so-called simulated deafness they should be considered not as isolated observations but within the context of the whole patient.

The patient complaining of a hearing impairment but found to have a serviceable acoustic receptor organ and no cerebral pathology may psychologically reject the sounds of society since they would obligate him. He may be withdrawing from responsibility, returning to a status of dependency, escaping from pressing reality. The deafness may also be deliberately designed for some material gain. Resolving such problems calls upon the resources of the otologist and the psychiatrist, the former to diagnose, clarify and classify the deafness, the latter to uncover the motivation.

Priest described his observations among military personnel. He reviewed and evaluated the many tests designed to study unilateral deafness. He emphasized the importance of examining the existence of unilateral deafness in military personnel, particularly when the patient denied the deafness, as well as exposing feigned unilateral deafness. He also defined the role of the otologist and that of the psychiatrist.

The tests for identifying deafness of nonorganic origin might be labeled "tests for the investigation of the complaint of deafness." Be it remembered that deafness is a symptom of disease, whether the pathology is organic or psychological or both.

Observation during the Interview

The observations begin when the patient first enters the physician's office. The otologist must be on the alert for clues of behavior, some of which may be gross, others minimal. The value of a patient's history depends not merely on what he says but how he says it, on his own interpretations and reactions to the chronological events he recites. One patient may appear overcomposed, another overanxious, another indifferent, another vague, another overexact. Clinical judgment is taxed to the utmost in the effort to evaluate properly such behavior.

The patient's history is explored in great detail. Some areas may be re-explored judiciously with different kinds of questions covering the same ground, possibly illuminating inconsistencies in the history. The physician can afford at least a benevolent skepticism of the complaint of any patient until he finds sufficient evidence to substantiate or doubt the patient's own opinions.

To cite some examples: A patient may complain that he cannot hear the telephone ring, yet when the otologist's phone rings the patient may promptly stop conversing. Or the patient may state that he hears only when he faces the speaker directly, but if the otologist is careless or clumsy enough to drop an article to the floor, as he stoops to retrieve it he may ask the patient a question which is answered without faltering. A patient who has never had any auditory rehabilitation may volunteer that he depends primarily on lip-reading (self-taught usually), yet understand a conversation with the otologist who talks with a cigarette between his lips. The otologist upon completing the history may leave the patient to enter the examining room, calling to the patient to follow him. Alacrity in response may further fortify the physician's suspicions. Hirsh states that the clinical tests of hearing depend on arbitrary conditioning of the moment. We have shown examples of the patient's conditioning for everyday situations. Such an approach is sounder and more reasonable psychologically than are recommendations suggesting that derogatory remarks be made in the patient's presence and his reactions noted, or that a coin be dropped to see whether the patient hears the sound of impact.

Patients with organic deafness tend to demonstrate behavioral patterns as the result of their deafness. In the presence of the doctor they will usually face him and be attentive to the purpose of the meeting. They may make an effort to hear, but this effort usually appears controlled and subtle.

In contrast, the patient alleging deafness, whether deliberately or unconsciously motivated, will often behave quite differently. He may sit down and assume an attitude as though he were unaware of the doctor's presence. He apparently is oblivious to the reason for this visit. The doctor may have to tap him to attract his attention, or remain ignored. Sometimes such patients will answer a question then turn away, so that with each question the patient demands some signal before he will pay attention to the doctor and attend to the next question.

Other patients may demonstrate exaggerated efforts to hear the doctor. They will draw up a chair and peer into the doctor's face, or each time the doctor addresses them they will throw their bodies forward as though to bridge the distance. Their efforts to hear are excessive, crude and elaborate. They may say they rely on lip reading, and may refuse to answer when the doctor obscures his face. However, they should be able to catch fragments of the conversation, and one can easily observe that the patient's eyes are leveled at the speaker's eyes and not at the speaker's lower face and lips.

Some of these patients may wear a hearing aid, from which certain clues may be abstracted. The ear mold may not fit the auricle properly. The patient may fumble when he attempts to remove the receiver and mold from his ear and when he tries to replace it. He may fail to turn off the hearing aid when he removes the receiver from his ear. Efficient constant hearing aid users invariably turn off the instrument before they remove the receiver from the ear in order to avoid the squeal of acoustic feed-back and to economize on battery drain. The inexperienced or untrained individual is unfamiliar with these small measures. Such patients expose their lack of good hearing aid habits.

Because such a person has serviceable unaided hearing, he usually turns the volume of the aid to a level which is comfortable for his relatively normal hearing. This amount of volume is insufficient for an individual who is as profoundly deafened as he alleges. All one has to do is to listen with the hearing aid at the volume setting at which the patient is using it to know that the volume is insufficent for a very deaf person.

If the doctor takes the aid from the patient he can inspect it to see if it shows evidence of usage and wear. A hearing aid which is in constant use will bear scratches and marks on the case and inside of the case from daily handling. An unused aid may appear brand new, or if the batteries have been left in the aid for a long time, the terminals may be corroded, and the case may be stained by a battery which has leaked.

The doctor can remove the batteries from the case and casually return the aid and the batteries to the patient. The experienced hearing aid user will assemble the parts deftly. Other patients may study how to insert the batteries, and by their awkward movements reveal their unfamiliarity with the aid.

Interrogating the patient about how he uses the aid may expose him further. How many hours a day and under what conditions does he use the aid. How long will the batteries last, the "A" battery, the "B" battery. What is the cost of the batteries singly, and what is the annual cost. Where does he buy the batteries. How often does the aid need repairs and what are the costs. What is the life of a hearing aid cord before it wears and breaks, and must be replaced. How many cords are used a year. The organically hard of hearing aid user is able to answer such questions promptly and accurately. The other patient may be no better informed than one unfamiliar with hearing aids.

The organically hard of hearing patient who uses a hearing aid and lip-reads efficiently will sometimes fail to hear exactly what has been said or will fail to understand. If a conversation is sufficiently lengthy he must fail occasionally in his acoustic and visual reception. Even with a hearing aid and expert lip reading, one cannot function with the same high efficiency as a normal-hearing person. If a person is suspected of feigning deafness and performs as efficiently as a normal hearing individual, never mistaking what is said to him, one may justifiably wonder if the patient's hearing is as poor as he alleges.

Out of his experience the doctor will learn to make use of certain words which are difficult for hard hearing persons to understand under their best listening conditions. When words like "illness" and "sickness" and others which are difficult to lip read are used during the course of conversation, the truly hard of hearing person may ask to have the sentence repeated, or may hesitate momentarily before replying as he tries to synthesize the meaning of the sentence. Other patients fail to demonstrate any difficulty in understanding these "difficult" words. They hear and understand more critically than most hard of hearing persons. They expose themselves by making mistakes of commission and omission.

Generally patients with monaural deafness demonstrate *astereophonia,* difficulty in localizing the source of a sound, and when addressed from an unanticipated quarter invariably gaze about in order to locate the speaker. The patient with non-organic monaural deafness fails to demonstrate the loss of localization of sound.

Another clue, a very important one, is the patient's speech patterns, as described by Penn. Invariably in the presence of long-standing binaural deafness, abnormalities of speech will appear, the variations depending on the duration of the deafness, its severity and its type. Of course, factors other than impaired acoustic function will modify one's speech, but development of speech impairment is a concomitant of binaural deafness. Speech of normal intensity, inflection and quality tends to contradict the allegation of bilateral deafness until adequate explanations may be found. Speech is the consort of hearing, and impairment of the latter often results in deterioration of its companion.

Clues during Clinical Examination

Upon performance of the otorhinolaryngological examination, further clues may be observed. The patient may readily obey instructions given him. During the mirror inspection of the larynx, the patient is asked to close his eyes and then is instructed to phonate so that the movements of the larynx may be noted. The instructions are given at a low conversational level. This examination is often sufficiently distracting to make the patient forget about his hearing; if his deafness is nonorganic he may obey the instructions given by the otologist at a voice volume which he apparently had been unable to hear during the history interview.

Exploration by Tests

By this time, the otologist will have obtained some impressions to be explored further by the various clinical tests of hearing. Often when preliminary observations have suggested that the hearing loss cannot be severe, the air conduction audiogram may demonstrate a most profound loss. There may be marked discrepancies between the audiograms of the two ears; the presumed worse ear may be better audiometrically than the presumed better ear. The audiometric curves may reveal bizarre configurations not ordinarily encountered in organic deafness. The bone conduction thresholds may also demonstrate unusual patterns.

If a continuous frequency audiometer is used, the following may sometimes be observed. When the loss of hearing appears to be most profound audiometrically, the physician sets the attenuator at about 50 decibles for 1000 cps. Then without altering the attenuator he rotates the frequency dial up to 4000 cps. If the patient signals that he hears the tone at the higher frequency but signals that he no longer hears the same tone after an interruption, there is evidence that he has heard at an intensity which he now denies. He had mistaken change of frequency for an apparent increase of loudness. This procedure can be repeated at lower intensities.

If the audiometry is performed by having the patient respond with the word "yes" each time he hears a tone, voice reactions may be observed. The moderately hard of hearing person and the normal hearing person usually will react with a change in voice volume to sudden wide fluctuations of intensity of the stimulus from the audiometer. If a patient alleging profound deafness responds with a loud "yes" to a tone of relatively great intensity and immediately with a soft "yes" to the same tone of much less intensity, the physician should infer that at some psychological level the patient has reacted to the changes of intensities which he has heard and recognized as being of different levels of loudness.

If the patient is observed during the testing through a one-way-vision window, not realizing that he is being watched, he may reveal by his facial and body reactions that he is restraining himself from responding or that he is in an anxiety-producing situation. If the patient uses the hand signal to indicate when he hears the tone, he may make small quivering movements of the fingers or hand, as though he is restraining himself from signaling while being aware of the tone. Many hard of hearing patients and normal subjects will demonstrate this kind of hesitating hand motion at threshold. The rate of eye blinking and the respiratory rate may change, indicating that the patient is aware of the stimulus, although he states that he does not hear the tone.

Repeating pure tone audiograms at intervals of several days may demonstrate that the thresholds of hearing vary considerably and that the findings are consistently inconstant.

Another test which explores hearing is the *speech-to-noise ratio test* described by Doerfler and Stewart. They observed that the normal-hearing ear is able to hear and understand speech at an intensity level less than that of measured masking noise simultaneously introduced with the speech. The truly hard of hearing ear usually will behave in a similar fashion. The patient with nonorganic deafness may state that he cannot hear the words because of the noise or object to a noise level of less intensity than that at which he had apparently been unable to hear speech. This indicates that he has heard less noise (in decibels) interfering with louder speech (in decibels) or he has heard the masking noise at an intensity which he previously had denied.

Another clue during the speech reception test is obtained when the patient responds with half syllables of the spondaic words (*see Chapter 11*). At other times such patients make up new words in response to the spondaic word stimulus. This kind of response, except in young children, mentally retarded patients, patients of foreign birth who speak and understand English poorly, and those with severe perceptive deafness, should make the observer suspicious of the patient's claims of acoustic impairment.

The *Lombard* test sometimes exposes or confirms binaural alleged deafness and also monaural alleged deafness. Masking noise, such as compressed air from the pressure suction apparatus usually found in a nose and throat office, introduced into both ears through a binaural stethoscope while the patient is reading aloud, often causes a variety of reactions. If hearing is normal or nearly so, most people will raise their voice volume in response to the masking of their hearing created by the noise in order to hear themselves read. Patients with nonorganic deafness may raise their voices or may read in a halting fashion or may mispronounce words. Occasionally the patient will drop the voice to an almost inaudible level. These patients may complain of pain or discomfort or demonstrate some evidence of distress or anxiety.

The Lombard test helps to confirm or uncover monaural deafness. The test may be performed in the following manner: While the patient reads aloud, masking noise is first introduced into the "deaf" ear. If there is an increase in voice volume, we give credence to the thought that the ear does hear. Even if the voice does not change, we then mask the better ear. If there is an increase in voice volume, we suspect that the "deafened" ear is impaired. If there is no change in voice volume when the good ear is masked, we suspect that the allegedly deafened ear is permitting the patient to monitor his own speech volume.

The *Stenger* test for unmasking of simulated monaural deafness can be performed with tuning forks in two ways. Usually the 512 decibel fork will suffice for the procedure. Two identical forks are used. The distance at which the good ear has heard the fork is obtained. The patient is blindfolded. Both forks are excited simultaneously. One fork is brought close to the alleged deaf ear, say to three inches. If the "bad" hears well, the fork applied to this ear will mask the hearing of the good ear so that it will not hear its own fork at the distance at which it previously did; the patient will therefore fail to indicate that he hears the fork with the good ear.

The Stenger phenomenon can be demonstrated with a binaurally normal hearing person. Two forks of the same frequency are excited at the same time. One fork is brought to about six inches from one ear. The subject states that he hears this fork. The second fork is then brought to within three inches from the other ear. The subject says that he no longer hears the first fork. The second fork is removed and the subject again hears the first fork.

The patient with significant monaural deafness when so tested will signal that at all times he hears the fork in the good ear. By contrast, the patient with monaural non-organic deafness will respond as does a binaurally normal hearing person.

The Stenger test can be performed with one tuning fork. The stem is inserted into a piece of rubber tubing about 3/8 inch in diameter and about thirty inches long. An olive tip is inserted into the other end of the tubing. The patient is instructed that he will inform the observer only when he hears the fork in the good ear. The patient is then blind-folded. The olive tip is inserted into the external meatus of the good ear and the fork is excited. The patient signals that he hears the tone in the good ear. The prongs of the fork are then brought close to the "bad" ear. If the bad ear hears the tone, it will mask the hearing of the good ear cerebrally, the sound source of which is thirty inches away via the tubing. The patient will necessarily signal that the good ear no longer hears the sound, thereby indicating that the "bad" ear hears. As an experiment, the reader can readily perform this test on himself.

The Stenger audiometry test requires more elaborate equipment, permitting more precise observations. One audiometer and two receivers, with an additional switch and

circuit before the phones, can be used. Two balanced audiometers, each with its own receiver, or a two-channel audiometer, are equally serviceable.

Usually the frequencies of 500, 1000, and 2000 cps. are
tested. The better ear will receive the tone at an intensity
level of about 15 decibels greater than its threshold. The
patient reports that he hears the tone in the good ear. The
same tone is then poured into the impaired ear at a level
of 15 decibels greater than that which the good ear is hearing. A patient with normal hearing will report that the
"good" ear, or the one which first heard the sound, no longer
hears it. When the tone to the second, or "bad" ear is interrupted, the patient reports that he hears the tone in the first
ear again. Actually, the two ears receive the same tone simultaneously although at two different intensities, the greater
intensity in the "bad" ear masking, cerebrally, the tone in
the better ear receiving the lower intensity. Patients with
organic monaural deafness will not succumb to this masking
until the intensity in the impaired ear is relatively large.
Patients with nonorganic monaural deafness will demonstrate the masking phenomenon. Two conclusions may then
be drawn: First, the alleged deafened ear does hear, and,
second, we know that the threshold for the particular frequency is no higher than the number of decibels which
masked the normal, or better, ear. For example, if 15 decibels
in the good normal ear is masked by 30 decibels in the
"deaf" ear, then the threshold of the "deaf" ear for a given
frequency can be no higher than 30 decibels and may be
lower (better). Testing the masking thresholds of the middle
three frequencies and determining that a positive Stenger
test is obtained at approximately serviceable hearing levels
for these frequencies is evidence of, at most, minimal acoustic
loss for the ear so tested.

The testing of hearing by *pure-tone audiometry with a*

psychogalvanometer offers one method whereby the cooperation of the patient by volitional signalling can be dispensed
with. Reasonably accurate audiometric pure-tone thresholds
can be elicited usually if technical, physical or mechanical
factors do not interpose artifacts or uncontrollable variables.
When reliable positive results are obtained, they can be
given as much credence as subjective tests. Interestingly,
many patients realizing that their hearing has been tested
"electrically" without any contribution on their part, as by
signaling, often give reasonably accurate subjective audiometric thresholds immediately thereafter.

8

TUNING FORKS AND BARS

Prior to the advent of the audiometer, tuning forks and other instruments were used for routine clinical testing of hearing. Tuning fork testing is still performed. Many hearing tests are identified by the names of those who introduced them. The *Schwabach* test compares the duration of bone conduction of the patient with the duration of the bone conduction of normal hearing. The *Weber* test is employed to ascertain the lateralization of sound by bone conduction. The *Rinne* test compares the duration of hearing by air conduction and by bone conduction. The *Gelle* test was conceived in an effort to determine the mobility of the stapes. The *Stenger* test is used to expose simulated monaural deafness.

The earlier tuning forks were made of steel. The low frequency forks were very heavy and unwieldy. Steel forks rust, which results in alterations in their acoustic characteristics. Often fingerprints become "etched" in the rust. Some forks were nickel-plated; when the plating peeled, adventitious sounds were produced.

Eventually aluminum alloy forks were developed.* Their weight is about one-third that of equivalent steel forks. They

---

* By the Riverbank Laboratories of Geneva, Ill.

are non-magnetic, unplated, non-rusting and non-tarnishing.
If given proper care they remain constant for many years.
Usually a case lined with soft fabric is furnished to protect
the forks from nicks or scratches. Misuse of forks or careless
handling, improper excitation will produce alterations in
their qualities and characteristics.

Aluminum alloy forks are made of bar stock of various
dimensions. Basically a tuning fork is a bar of metal, presenting two prongs blending into a common stem. When the
fork is excited the prongs vibrate transversely and the stem
longitudinally. The size and weight of the bar or fork de-
termines its frequency.

When a fork vibrates the tone is emitted from several
surfaces of the prongs: from the external sides, the lateral
sides, the edges where these sides meet, and from the tips.
The prongs vibrate with a wide amplitude of lesser intensity compared with the stem which vibrates with less
amplitude but greater intensity. The edges produce the
least intensity, the tips generate a greater intensity, and the
lateral and outer surfaces propagate still greater and about
equal intensities. Early measurements suggested that the intensity produced by the outer surfaces of the prong may be
slightly greater than that emitted by the sides.

These variations of intensities can readily be demonstrated. Hold the fork by the stem and excite it. Bring the
prong close to the ear and present the several surfaces to be
heard by air conduction. Holding the fork vertically, rotate
it slowly: the loudness will vary appreciably. If an edge of
a prong is held at an optimum angle in relation to the ear,
very little sound will be heard. If the fork is then rotated
only slightly the loudness will increase considerably.

It follows that the manner of presentation of the forks is
an important factor, and when testing hearing the forks
should always be presented uniformily and in a constant

manner. The outer surface of a prong should be turned toward the auricle when testing for air conduction.

Forks may be of two types, either of single vibrations or of double vibrations. It is necessary to distinguish between the two, as the difference between similar forks of single vibrations and double vibrations is a whole octave.

The better sets of forks are, perhaps, the Hartman series of five forks ranging from 128 dv to 2048 dv, and the Edelman set of eight forks ranging from 16 dv to 4096 dv. Some otologists also include the two Bezold forks; the unweighted 108 dv usually being used for the Weber and Schwabach tests, and the 435 dv for Rinne testing.

The contemporary aluminum alloy forks are available in several sets: class A 1, class A 2 and A 2M, and class A 3 and A 3M. The letter M designates the medical sets of forks. The forks can be tuned to a choice of pitches: International, Concert, and Physical Scientific for research. When ordering forks it is important to state which tuning is preferred.

Class A 1. Matched set No. 1 consists of seven forks comprising the seven C octaves from 64 cps to 4096 cps. Matched set No. 2 consists of thirteen forks comprising the chromatic octaves about middle C, tuned to either International or Concert pitch. These forks are made of ½"x1½" bar stock. The stems are threaded and fitted permanently into hard rubber handles which prevents transmission of heat from the hand to the fork.

Class A 2. Matched set No. 1 consists of seven forks comprising the seven C octaves from 64 cps to 4096 cps. Matched set No. 2 consists of thirteen forks comprising the chromatic octaves about middle C tuned to either International or Concert pitch.

The stems of class A 2M are appoximately three and one half inches long, about one inch longer than the same forks without the M designation.

Class A 3. Matched set No. 1 consists of seven forks comprising the seven C octaves from 64 cps to 4096 cps. They are made of ⅜" x 1" bar stock. The M set has a stem about ¼ inch longer, making the stem about two inches in length.

The forks are easily excited to large amplitudes and the following methods of excitation are recommended by the manufacturer: *C-64 to C-256,* strike the prong with a soft rubber hammer or on the heel of the hand. *C-256 to C-1024,* strike with a medium hard rubber hammer. *C-1024* and above, strike with a hard rubber hammer or with a soft wooden mallet.

Tuning bars—class AB—are available for classroom instruction and demonstration, when a precision frequency source of long audible time and of large initial amplitude is desired. Bars can be obtained tuned to any frequency from 4000 cps (approximately 25" x 11/16") to 25000 cps (approximately 3" x 5/8"). The frequency is marked on the sleeve of each bar.

Clinical Testing with Tuning Forks

To test hearing clinically with tuning forks two desiderata need be fulfilled: qualitative measurement of hearing, and quantitative measurement. The qualitative requirement is met by the true fundamental frequency of a fork produced by a reliable manufacturer.

One method of calibrating a fork quantitatively is to excite it to its maximum and, with a normal-hearing ear, listen to it until it can no longer be heard. The number of seconds elapsed until the *decay* (decreasing loudness) arrives at an inaudible point can be determined with a stopwatch. Several runs with normal-hearing ears, both for air conduction and for bone conduction, will allow for quantitative calibrations in seconds. The number of seconds less which another ear hears the tone as compared to the "normal" calculations is a measure of the hearing loss.

Another means of calibrating a fork quantitatively is to measure its maximum intensity with a sound level meter and follow its rate of decay in time until it can no longer be heard by a normal-hearing ear. Since the rate of decay is fairly uniform, the rate per second of decrement may be estimated.* For example, if a fork's maximum intensity is 100 decibels and it becomes inaudible to a normal-hearing ear, at a presumed threshold of zero decibel, in 100 seconds, then the average rate of decay may be considered to be one decibel per second. If this fork should be heard by another ear for only 40 seconds, the threshold of hearing for the ear at the frequency of the fork is 60 decibels. Thus, forks might be calibrated both for air conduction and for bone conduction.

When testing with forks certain considerations should be entertained. It is preferable to test the hearing under controlled environmental conditions, which already have been described. A fork should always be excited the same way. Generally the lower-tuned forks should be stimulated with softer implements than the higher-tuned forks. Some uniformity of stimulation has been obtained with the use of a pendulum: a rubber weight is permitted to fall through a measured arc and strike the fork. The percussion center of a fork is about at the junction of the first and second thirds of the prong, and it is this zone which should receive the impact of the exciting blow.

---

* The rate of decrement of forks varies directly with their frequencies. The rate of decrement of the lower frequencies is from 0.25 decibels to 1 decibel per second. The higher frequency fork's rate of decrement is from 2 to 4 decibels per second. When a fork is used to test bone conduction, the rate of decrement is more rapid because it is damped when the shank is pressed against the head.

A fork should be excited to its maximum vibration. Overtones may be produced but these promptly become dissipated as the fork settles down to its fundamental. The outer surface of the prong should be brought close to the auricle, and always to the same distance from the auricle. Care must be exercised that the fork does not touch the patient, as such contact will damp the fork. The patient is asked to report whenever he hears the tone, and when he does so, the fork is removed, then returned to the ear. This is repeated until the patient no longer hears the fork.

The reason for removing the fork from the ear when it has been heard is to relieve the ear from continuous acoustic exposure to the stimulus, which will produce auditory fatigue. If the ear fatigues it will become insensitive to the minimal stimuli to which it might respond at threshold, and false, raised, thresholds will be recorded. This precaution also should be observed when bone conduction testing is performed. The stem of the fork should be placed against the mastoid process, then removed and replaced repeatedly until the sound is no longer heard.

The use of tuning forks to determine the presence of monaural deafness of non-organic origin, as well as to validate monaural organic deafness, has been described in *Chapter 7* in the discussion of the Stenger Test.

9

TINNITUS

The most common symptom associated with impaired hearing is tinnitus; noises in the ears or in the head. Some patients are more distressed by these noises than by their hearing difficulties. Many patients complain primarily of head noises, and may have no handicapping acoustic impairment.

Tinnitus in the presence of serviceable hearing is encountered among individuals who demonstrate a discrete or focal hearing loss, such as is observed following exposure to gun fire. The high tone perceptive deafness of presby-acusia may not be great enough to cause any significant impaired acoustic reception, but the associated tinnitus may prove most distressing. These are two examples among a host of others in which head noises may be the dominant symptom, and in which the acoustic spectral defect may be inconsequential.

Patients often state that the loudness of the tinnitus is so great that it interferes with their ability to hear normal speech; or that the noises are loud enough to disturb ability to concentrate and work, and to interrupt sleep.

If the loudness of the patient's tinnitus is measured it often appears to be within a few decibels of the patient's threshold of hearing. If the patient's hearing loss is slight, the measured loudness of the tinnitus may not be great. If the hearing loss is profound, the "loudness" so measured may be marked. But the apparent loudness as experienced by the patient seems to be a relative thing. Some patients complain that the tinnitus is very loud and the measurements reveal that the intensity in decibels is not large. The measured intensities of other patients are significantly great, nevertheless they may not be unduly disturbed by what appears to be considerably loud, and apparently should be subjectively loud. The sensation of loudness of the tinnitus is a subjective psychological phenomenon.

At times the tinnitus may be studied quantitatively and qualitatively. If a patient has monaural deafness and monaural tinnitus it is possible to compare the tones of the audiometer introduced into the normal ear with the sounds which the patient experiences in the affected ear. The frequencies of the audiometer are introduced into the normal ear one after the other until the patient states that one of the frequencies sounds similar to his subjective noises. Then with the attenuator the intensity of this frequency is altered until the patient thinks that the subjective noise and the audiometer tone seem equally loud. Presumably the findings are a measure of the patient's tinnitus.

Binaural tinnitus may be more difficult to match. It is feasible to try to mask the tinnitus with an audiometric tone similar to the patient's subjective noises. The frequency may be identifiable, and possibly the loudness may also be matched. It also may be feasible to mask the tinnitus with the masking noise of the audiometer, and consider that the amount of masking just necessary to obliterate the tinnitus is a measure of the loudness of the tinnitus. Some patients have discovered for themselves that they are able to mask their tinnitus when they try to fall asleep by playing the radio softly next to their bed. Patients also notice that when the ambient noise is sufficiently loud they no longer hear the head noises. Of course the ambient noise is usually in excess of 35 decibels. It has also been observed that the tinnitus may become inaudible when a hearing aid is worn, although this is not consistently so with all hearing aid wearers.

Often tinnitus begins apparently spontaneously long after the deafness has been established. The duration of the tinnitus may be short, hours or a few days, or it may become firmly established. In other instances tinnitus of many years duration has subsided suddenly and has remained inaudible for years, and apparently permanently.

Healthy people with no otic or acoustic history of any kind experience sudden bursts of tinnitus, often high pitched, of momentary duration. Furthermore most people with no aural defects have experienced tinnitus when they are in a very quiet environment, where the ambient noise is considerably reduced.

Comparative Study of Tinnitus

Because these have been the experiences among normal people with normal ears, a study was undertaken to determine whether tinnitus can be observed among normals, and to compare their observations with the tinnitus described by patients with aural pathology and functional impairment.

A sound-proof chamber was used. The ambient noise level was probably between 15 and 18 decibels. Exact measurements could not be made due to the limitations of the sound level meters at hand.

Eighty adults, apparently normally hearing males and females, from 18 to 60 years of age were included. The selection was predicated on a denial of past or present aural disease. They reported no deafness or tinnitus, and considered themselves in good health. They were representatives of a sedentary population, including physicians, dentists, teachers, students, administrators, clerks and housewives.

Upon entering the sound-proof room the subjects were instructed to make notes of sounds which might be detected. No suggestion was given that the source of sound might be within the subject himself. The time of observation was usually limited to five minutes or less. Written details of their observations were obtained. Seventy-five subjects, 94 per cent, experienced sound. From these reports it appears that tinnitus is present constantly but is masked by the ambient noise which floods our environment. This ambient noise level for ordinary quiet living conditions usually exceeds 35 decibels, and apparently is of sufficient intensity to mask physiological tinnitus which remains subaudible.

The control group was composed of one-hundred hard-of-hearing patients, consecutively admitted veterans of military service. Their histories, otorhinological examinations, and pure tone audiograms were obtained. A diagnosis of deafness and its type was recorded. Head noises, tinnitus, was a com-

TABLE 1. Diagnosis of Deafness and Incidence of Tinnitus in 100 Patients.

Diagnosis	Number of Patients	Tinnitus		No Tinnitus
		Constant	Inconstant	
Conductive deafness without otosclerosis	20	3	10	7
Otosclerosis (1 case mixed deafness, 7 cases conductive deafness)	8	4	4	0*
Perceptive deafness	55	21	18	16
Mixed deafness	8	2	5	1
Mixed deafness of one ear, perceptive deafness of other	5	3	1	1
Diagnosis not available	4	2	0	2
	100	35	38	27

* In a larger group of 83 otosclerotic patients in our clinic, 85 per cent had tinnitus and 15 per cent were free of it.

plaint of 73 per cent of these patients. The loss of hearing
of each of these patients was of sufficient severity to warrant
the recommendation and use of a hearing aid and a course
of auditory rehabilitation. *See Table 1.*

A total of 39 different sounds were described by both
groups. Of these, 27 sounds were named in the impaired
group, and 23 sounds in the normal group. While a majority
in both groups reported hearing only one sound, a substan-
tial number of persons in each group distinguished two or
more sounds. The sounds described as "ring," "hum" and
"buzz" were enumerated most frequently in both groups,
comprising about 50 per cent of the responses of each group.
Eleven sounds recorded were identified in both groups.

Sounds Recorded by Patients and Normal Group

(Patients' totals listed first):

Ring	32–11	Falling water	3– 4
Hum	10–16	Roar	5– 2
Buzz	12–13	Hiss	3– 3
Whistle	9– 3	Airplane	2– 1
Insects, crickets	2– 6	Zooming-whizzing	1– 2
		Tap	1– 1

Sounds Recorded by Normal Group Only:

Steam	4	Rushing	1
Bell	3	Singing	1
Click	3	Musical sound	1
Fog horn	2	Machinery	1
Sea shell	2	Rumble	1
Heart beat	2	Hollow sound	1
Drone	1	Squeal	1
Truck	1	Echo	1

Sounds Recorded by Patients Only:

Pulse	7	Surf	1
Thumping pulsation	4	Vibration	1
Squeak	3	Throbbing	1
Watch tick	2	Rubbing cloth	1
Pressure	2	Rustling leaves	1
Tunnels	2	Stuffiness	1

Categories of Tinnitus

As considered here, *tinnitus aurium* is a medical term describing sounds of physiological or pathological origin, which may or may not always be perceived in consciousness.

Kerrison enumerated five general groups of sounds: (1) *obstructive;* (2) *circulatory*—vascular alterations; (3) *labyrinthine*—cochlear sounds; (4) *neurotic*—instability of the auditory nerve; (5) *cerebral sounds*—involvement of the auditory centers.

Fowler has divided tinnitus into two categories: (1) *vibratory,* mechanical, exogenus—factual sounds within the body, and (2) *non-vibratory,* biochemical endogenous—total absence of sound outside the body.

Vibratory tinnitus is real sound of a physical source such as muscle activity, or vascular alteration. Non-vibratory tinnitus is nonfactual sound: an illusion of sound caused by an irritation of the auditory neural elements. The points of origin may be anywhere from the tympanic promontory, along the pathways to the cortex inclusive.

Atkinson also has divided tinnitus into two categories; extrinsic and intrinsic, which appear to include the two types already mentioned. He considers intrinsic tinnitus as an auditory paresthesia, a paresthesia of the auditory nerve, of vascular origin and to be so treated.

Wegel recorded: "Tinnitus is a pathologic symptom . . . I am under the impression that the presence of tinnitus . . . generally indicates an active or progressive lesion and that the cessation of it . . . is an indication that the degeneration or atrophy of tissue has been arrested." But then he continued, "people entirely without tinnitus are extremely rare, if such cases exist at all."

In 1941 Fowler wrote, "It has been found that the presence of tinnitus is always associated with more or less deafness." In 1944 he altered this view, writing: "It may be, and often is, present in some form in persons who have no apparent aural or other disease."

Kopetzky stated that tinnitus is a symptom signifying disturbed sensation, a symptom of aural disease. He continued that tinnitus may appear before symptomatic deafness.

Lempert suggested on the basis of his observations associated with middle ear surgery that "tonus impulses originating in the sensory fibers of the trigeminus, the sympathetic, or glossopharyngeal may enter the tympanic plexus, but normally are not heard." In selected cases, he recommended tympanosympathectomy.

Fowler further described tinnitus, of which the patient is consciously aware, as "audible," and tinnitus not ordinarily impinging on the consciousness as "subaudible." He found tinnitus in 86 per cent of 200 patients. He indicated that subaudible tinnitus must be sought for by examination. He also determined that the loudness of tinnitus was within 5 to 10 decibels above threshold. Tinnitus may be measured for frequency, loudness and quality. It may be a single frequency or multiple frequencies and difficulties may be encountered in its identification. The exact loudness may also be difficult to determine. Fowler described techniques for making such measurements.

Audible tinnitus at times appears to interfere with hearing. Patients often state that were it not for their head noises their hearing would be better, and that when the head noises are louder the deafness is more severe. It does not necessarily follow that the tinnitus is always responsible for this. Possibly with increased deafness the head noises are less easily masked and so appear louder subjectively. Fowler has described the "busy line" effect, whereby receptor cells and neural pathways already preoccupied by an intrinsic stimulus are not receptive to an external stimulus.

Tinnitus in Disease

Some conditions in which audible tinnitus has been observed are:

(1) Otosclerosis.

(2) Ménière's disease.

(3) Lermoyez's syndrome.

(4) Pressure or neuritis of the auditory apparatus; brain tumor, eighth nerve tumor, aneurysm.

(5) Otitis media; acute, chronic, suppurative, nonsuppurative.

(6) Otitis interna; acute, chronic.

(7) Deafness; conductive, perceptive, mixed.

(8) Normal hearing with discrete frequency defect.

(9) Nasopharyngeal diseases; eustachian salpingitis, sinusitis, pharyngitis, mucosal hypertrophy, hyperplasia, tumor, infection of lymphoid tissue.

(10) Dental pathology; malocclusion, malfunction of temporomandibular joint, impaction, infection.

(11) Myositis; cervical, pharyngeal, tympanic.

(12) Intoxication—drug; quinine, alcohol, salicylates, caffeine, tobacco, antiluetic agents, streptomycin, thyroid gland extract.

(13) Intoxication—systemic; gastrointestinal, foci of infection.

(14) Allergy.

(15) Cardiovascular pathology; blood dyscrasias, anemia, hypertension, hypotension, vascular anomalies, arteriosclerosis, cardiac diseases.

(16) Metabolic dysfunction; thyroidism, water balance disturbances.

(17) Trauma; acoustic, acute.

(18) Trauma; acoustic, chronic.

(19) Systemic fatigue.

(20) Momentary tinnitus, spontaneous (idiopathic).

(21) Impacted cerumen.

(22) Cervical constriction.

(23) Psychoses.

(24) Otic herpes.

(25) Bell's palsy.

(26) Foreign body trauma to the ear.

(27) Head injury; concussion, postconcussion syndrome.

(28) Myringitis.

(29) Hemorrhage; tympanum or myringa.

Treatment of Tinnitus

The ideal approach to the treatment of audible tinnitus would seem to be a therapeutic assault on the related etiological factors. At present there is no sure way to accomplish this. Frequently the etiological agent no longer exists, the tinnitus, however, persists. Some of the contemporary measures are:

Medical:

(1) Medication; bromides, barbiturates, other sedatives, potassium iodide, vitamins, benzyl cinnamate, antiallergic drugs, histamine therapy, intravenous procaine.

(2) Local therapy to disease processes.

(3) Elimination of drugs and intoxicants.

(4) Elimination of foci of infection.

(5) Correction of faulty gastrointestinal function.

(6) Correction of metabolic diseases.

(7) Control of diseases of the vascular system and blood forming organs.

(8) Dietary control of fluids, salt, and water balance.

(9) Dental rehabilitation.

(10) Intratympanic medication.

(11) Therapy directed to correct nose and throat pathology, including roentgen and radium therapy.

(12) Politzerization, inflation, massage.

(13) Removal of cerumen.

(14) Psychotherapy.

(15) Hearing aid.

(16) Electrical therapies, i.e., ultra violet, quartz lamps, galvanism.

Surgical:

(1) Otologic; ossiculectomy, mastoidectomy, chorda tympani resection, fenestration of the labyrinth, obliteration of the saccus endolymphaticus.

(2) Rhinologic.

(3) Spinal tap.

(4) Cranial surgery for tumor, vascular anomalies, section of eighth cranial nerve. Stellate ganglion block.

(5) Splanchnectomy and similar technics for alleviation of hypertension.

It would appear, then, that tinnitus will not be eliminated by any treatment but at best can only become subaudible. This, of course, would be welcomed both by the patient and the physician.

Fowler has emphasized the value of explaining to the patient the nature of his tinnitus: that it is a symptom and not a disease, and that despite its annoying and distressing presence, it does not imply a threat to him. An understanding of the symptom and a recognition of its relative significance in some instances may reconcile the sufferer to his burden.

INFANTS AND CHILDREN

The anamnesis of these little patients has already been mentioned in some detail in *Chapter 4*. One should explore the prenatal, parturient, neonatal and subsequent episodes in the life of the patient. The maternal history is included because of its intimate relationship to that of the fetus.

The baby's development is studied to learn the nature of his physical and mental growth. Has the child attempted to sit, crawl, stand, walk at the appropriate ages; if he is old enough has toilet training been accomplished? What are the feeding habits, ability to dress himself; is his sleeping apparently normal or disturbed? What is his general behavior; active, lethargic, or hyperactive? Are there temper tantrums or rocking or head banging? How does he communicate to make his demands known: by calling, by gestures, or does he fail to make demands?

Initial Observations

During the early stages of the investigation it may be well to permit the child freedom of movement about the office. If the child is old enough he should be given the opportunity to explore the environs of the office if he wants to. Clues may be obtained by his behavior: how he relates to the over-all situation, to the office personnel, to the toys which are offered to him, to those sounds about the office which may be different from those to which he is accustomed at home; whether he responds when the office telephone rings, or makes an effort to play with the phone or tries to answer it. A member of the office staff may manipulate several of the noise makers without being seen by the child. Does the child react to these noises and does he seek the source of their origin?

Toys, jig-saw puzzles and books should be made available to the child. Does he demonstrate interest or indifference, is his interest sustained or is his attention span momentary, does he accept one toy to the exclusion of the others and persevere in playing with it? While he is occupied with the toys, the noise instruments can again be sounded, and observations can be made whether the child is at all respon-sive to the acoustic stimuli. The otologist may play with the toys, possibly teaching the child to build a tower of blocks. Will the child attempt to imitate such suggestions or be in-different? The otologist may begin to gain the child's friend-ship and favor by such playing and may also formulate some idea of the child's mental scope and emotional function. During such play the manual dexterity is noted as well as the handedness.

From these observations one may gain some idea as to how readily the child may be tested. A very lethargic child may be unresponsive to the testing and a hypomanic child will not remain quiet long enough to be tested. Usually the patient rather than the physician will set the pace of the functional examination.

Diagnostic Considerations

There are several broad diagnostic considerations to be distinguished:

(1) organic deafness

(2) organic brain damage

(3) mental retardation

(4) psychiatric disturbances

(5) a combination of organic deafness with any of these other defects.

In a survey by Kastein and Fowler, 150 children and infants were observed for acoustic function because of impaired, delayed or absent speech. Fifty per cent of these patients demonstrated some cerebral or psychological disease in which there was no deafness. One third of the patients demonstrated organic deafness and the remainder had a diagnosis of organic deafness with brain damage, or with mental retardation, or with emotional disturbance. It is apparent that when a patient from this early age group is studied because of the failure of development of normal speech, there is as much chance that the etiology is some pathological process other than that of otic pathology with deafness. Furthermore, among these children who have deafness, a significant number will also demonstrate some other disease, of cerebral, intellectual or emotional etiology.

The otologist, therefore, may elect to recommend that the child be studied neurologically and psychologically before any further testing of acoustic function. Some other process may be found and reveal whether the child does or does not appear to hear. The otologist will then be better prepared to determine in what manner he can proceed to study the acoustic function of the patient.

Methods and Situations of Testing

Various noise-producing instruments have been described by Utley. They range from low frequency tom-toms (60 cps) and tambourines to high frequency bells (6200 cps). These instruments can be calibrated by the use of an oscillograph, beat frequency oscillator, and sound level meter. The frequencies can be measured, and also the intensities at various distances. If calibration equipment is not readily available, a tester who has normal hearing may be able to make a relatively rough estimate of the output by matching the frequencies and the intensities with the frequencies of the audiometer. This is a much less exact method of measuring the sound production of the instruments, but still is of some value. If a child responds to the noise makers of the lower frequencies but not to those of the higher frequencies, an estimate of the width of the auditory spectrum may be obtained. By varying the distance between the child and the instruments which he apparently hears, some quantitative estimates can also be approximated.

Over a period of months it may be noted that a child's acuity of hearing appears to have increased. This may be accounted for by the learning experiences of the patient. With growth and increasing familiarity with sounds, he will heed and attend to sounds of lesser intensities than he had at an earlier age when he was less aware of the existence and importance of sound.

If the patient can be made to understand that a game will be played, pure tone audiometry can be performed. The child is informed that he will listen to a telephone represented by the air conduction receiver; or that he is an "airplane pilot." Each time he hears a sound in the phone he should ring a bell, such as a cowbell, which has been offered him for this purpose. If the child understands the game he may be most cooperative and reasonably exact with his responses.

Another means of gaining the child's interest is to teach him to build a tower of blocks. He is taught that each time he hears the tone he is to place a toy block on top of another. He can then be taught to remove the blocks each time he hears a tone. In this manner pure tone audiometry may be accomplished at least for the range of the speech frequencies.

It may also be possible to perform speech reception threshold tests. Several toys (whose designations are spondaic words —*see Chapter 11, Table 2*) are placed before the child. Either with the phones or with the free field speaker, a live voice instructs the child; "pick up the *toothbrush*," "where is the *airplane*," "show me the *baseball*." This kind of testing is effective in determining the presence of serviceable hearing, particularly if parents have been in doubt. It may also help to uncover the presence of unilateral hearing impairment.

The technique of psychogalvanic skin response audiometry has been described in *Chapter 5*. The electrodes of the galvanometer may be affixed to the infants foot and the stimulating electrodes to another extremity. The baby is held in the mother's lap and is kept gently preoccupied in the effort to have him remain quiet and relatively immobile. A pediatric dose of a sedative may be orally administered about one hour before the tests are performed. The sedation usually does not interfere with the responses. The mother can hold the receiver close to the baby's ear during the test.

Usually two members of the testing staff cooperate; one performs the test and operates the equipment and the other observes the child for random movements which stimulate the galvanometer producing spurious fluctuations of the needle. As with adults, some tests are performed with ease and reliable results are obtained; at other times no conclusions may be forthcoming.

Children between the ages of two and five may prove more difficult to test with the galvanometer. Just as in all their other waking periods they move about continuously, and usually will not remain sufficiently inactive for successful use of the test. If, however, the child is permitted to play with toys at a table, he may be passive enough to permit testing.

Children with brain damage, such as those with cerebral palsy, should have hearing tests performed on them, as part of the physical examination. The more severely involved patients may be unable to manipulate the toys, but the noise makers or audiometer may be used effectively to learn if the patient responds to sounds.

Let us turn to the otolaryngological examination. Many children may have had several examinations elsewhere and may have developed an antipathy to further examinations and to all that the white gown, head mirror and instruments mean to them. For this reason it is often better to postpone the performance of the physical examination until most of the functional studies have been accomplished, before the patient becomes too unruly to submit gracefully to them.

Tests of the function of the stato-kinetic end organs should be included as a part of the physical examination. Usually stimulation of the equilibratory labyrinth with cold water is an effective test. If the cold stimulation provokes a response there will be ocular nystagmus and the child may sway to one side, or if permitted to walk he may stagger. The direction of the nystagmus and the direction of the sway of the body, with normal functioning labyrinths, will be in accordance with known physiological observations.

The labyrinths can also be stimulated by seating an adult,

usually a parent, in a Barany rotating chair, and then seating the patient on the parent's lap. Both are rotated, and the child is examined at the end of rotation. If the labyrinths are active, nystagmus is observed and the baby may fall to one side, in the direction of the slow component of the nystagmus. This test should be performed with some circumspection as the adult may be stimulated more than the patient.

Unresponsive labyrinths are indicative of their nonfunction and highly suggestive that profound perceptive deafness also is present. A nonfunctioning labyrinth may also be observed in very severe monaural perceptive deafness, at any age. With some evidence of appreciable loss of hearing in an infant, the lack of function of the equilibratory end organs is a confirmation that these sensory structures have been extensively damaged. The presence of normal functioning equilibratory end organs does not preclude the possibility that the inner ears are impaired acoustically. Nevertheless it is important to know and record whether the peripheral equilibratory system does function normally or not, and to know also if the patient has the additional handicap in the loss of these other very important sensory structures.

Another step in the examination consists of roentgen studies of the tympanic and petrosal anatomy. X-ray examinations can delineate the tympanum, semicircular canals, and cochlea. Occasionally some of these structures may not be identified by x-ray projections, which may suggest that the structures have failed to develop, additional confirmatory evidence of organic defect.

Here as in all medicine the whole patient is viewed. Having determined by the history, the physical examination, and the functional examinations that the infant is deaf, plans will be made so that his education, particularly acoustic training and speech training, will be begun promptly. It is important that maximum use be made of whatever residual hearing remains. The child must learn that he lives in a world of sound, and that sound is meaningful. The educational process is a lengthy one but can produce an adult able to communicate with his fellows and to lead a happy productive life.

11

SPEECH AUDIOMETRY

Accurate assessment of the ability to hear and understand spoken material had its origins in the practical studies of workers in telephonic and wartime communications equipment. Syllable, word and sentence lists were constructed for the purpose of evaluating the relative ability of communication systems to pass speech signals. It was then a logical development to adapt this speech test material for use in hearing measurement. That otologists had a need for testing hearing for speech is clearly evident in the long-standing use of the whispered and voice distance fraction test.

Uncalibrated Live Voice

The distance fraction test, while an expression of this need, is riddled with too many weaknesses to be considered a satisfactory testing tool. Since the test is almost never performed in an adequately sound treated room, little reliance can be placed upon it because the inverse square law of sound pressure does not obtain. The intensity of the spoken words at the listener's head then is vaguely defined, depending not only on the speaker but also on the reflections of sound from the walls, ceiling and floor. Accurate measurement is further vitiated by the wide fluctuation in intensity of a given speaker's voice, let alone the variations from one speaker to another. Other difficulties are introduced by the failure to use standardized material, lack of masking in unilateral deafness, etc. Many an individual with perceptive deafness but with fairly intact hearing for the low frequencies has been suspected of malingering because of his ability to understand some directions given at a certain distance, followed by failure to repeat all words spoken at a lesser distance.

The pure tone audiometer possesses inherent quantitative advantages over the tuning fork and allows wider scope in testing. Speech audiometry likewise is quantitatively superior to the distance fraction test and broadens the range of exploration.

4 C Numbers Test

A word might be said at this point concerning the Western Electric phonograph audiometer which is widely used in school systems as a screening instrument. Developed in its original form almost thirty years ago, this audiometer is somewhat akin to modern speech audiometry as regards presentation of speech. The test items used are composed of the digits one, two, three, four, five, six and eight. An individual with loss of hearing for just the high frequencies, might recognize the vowel differences that would enable him to score sufficiently high to pass this screening test. Recent careful investigations have demonstrated the inadequacies of the Western Electric "fading numbers" test as a screening device.

Speech Reception Threshold

The pure tone audiometer uses average normal hearing

as the reference level. The ratio, in decibels, between the measured threshold and the normal or zero line, is taken to be the hearing loss at a given frequency. A similar concept obtains with regard to the speech reception threshold. If selected material is heard by the normal ear at zero decibels, and by a defective ear at 40 decibels, then the defective ear has a 40 decibel loss of hearing for speech.

A good deal of work has gone into the selection and preparation of speech material for use in testing hearing. The pioneer work was done at the Bell Telephone Laboratories. Major achievements were recorded during World War II studies at Harvard University's Psycho-Acoustic Laboratory, with succeeding refinements at the Central Institute for the Deaf. The loss of hearing for speech (speech reception threshold) is related to the loss of hearing for pure tones (pure tone threshold). Both tests seek to make a fundamental quantitative measurement. In selecting words, therefore, it was considered important that they be familiar in the language, in order to minimize the importance of the factors of intelligence and knowledge of vocabulary.

It is of essential importance in speech threshold measurement that the words used be alike in their difficulty of audibility. Some types of words have much higher homogeneity of audibility than do others. It was found that the test criteria were best met in words of the spondee stress pattern (two-syllable words equally accented). These have uniformly higher audibility than do monosyllables or unselected disyllabic words. When both of the syllables receive stress, there is greater ease of audition (more clues are presented) than in the case of monosyllabic words or two-syllable words in which only one syllable is stressed.

A number of testing benefits accrue by reason of the uniformity of audibility possessed by the eighty-four spondaic words which were chosen. It follows from what has been said that these words will be equally audible in a narrow range of intensity. In testing a hard of hearing patient, the level at which he hears correctly one word out of five presented should be relatively close to the level at which he understands four of the five words. This "steepness of function" makes for precision and speed in pinpointing the speech reception threshold. The homogeneity and ease of audibility of the spondees has resulted in their bearing a fairly close correlation to audibility of connected speech, and the latter represents the kind of conversational demands that make up the bulk of an individual's everyday auditory activity.

The *Harvard Spondaic Words* were prepared at the Harvard University Psycho-Acoustic Laboratory in phonograph recordings in two arrangements. Auditory Test No. 9 is recorded so that forty-two words are disposed in seven groups, each group containing six words. As the test record proceeds from group to group, there is a decrease of 4 decibels in the intensity level of each group of six words. Thus the final group of six words on each record is 24 decibels weaker than the first group on the record. In Auditory Test No. 14 seventy spondees are recorded at a uniform intensity.

Discrimination Testing

Once threshold has been determined, valuable diagnostic information can then be obtained by speech tests at levels above threshold. Measurements at these supra-liminal levels are designed to explore how a defective ear operates when its hearing loss for speech is overridden by presenting material at a sufficiently intense level. What is sought is a measure of how well the ear can discriminate. The normal ear, with a speech reception threshold of zero decibels, performs in a certain manner at the 40 decibel level. How does a defective ear with a speech reception threshold of 25 decibels perform at the 65 decibel level? An ear may deviate to the extent of an elevated threshold but with relative normalcy above threshold, or it may be deviant for both threshold and levels well above threshold.

To test for this function, it was found best to construct other groups of word lists. These are the phonetically balanced or PB word lists. They consist of familiar words of one syllable arranged in groupings of fifty words to a list. The intention is that each list be of comparable difficulty, and of equal phonetic structure. Aside from some practical compromises, the lists contain the elements or sounds spoken in the frequency of their occurrence in the language. The words were read to normal hearing subjects and those words which were at the extremes of easy and difficult audibility were eliminated.

The product of the research at the Psycho-Acoustic Laboratory was offered to clinical examiners of hearing and auditory impairment. Twenty PB lists, each containing fifty words, also were made available. This allowed for testing with lists which were constructed so that test score differences could be allotted to factors other than differences in the equality of the word lists.

Lists of the Central Institute for the Deaf

Clinical experience in the years following World War II indicated that some of the Harvard test words, such as "mote" and "bon bon," are not as familiar as is desirable for test purposes. Accordingly, a project was established at the Central Institute for the Deaf (C.I.D.) St. Louis, Missouri, with a view to correcting this difficulty. In addition, the PB lists were reconstructed in an effort to achieve better phonetic balance. From the original Harvard tests and PB lists were derived C.I.D. Auditory Test W-1 and W-2 and four PB lists identified as C.I.D. Auditory Test W-22.*

In addition to improvement of the test items, it was intended that standardized disc recordings be made commercially available for clinical use.

Spondaic Words

C.I.D. Auditory Test W-1 consists of thirty-six spondaic words (Table 2). Six lists, A, B, C, D, E, F were prepared with rearrangement of the word order. For each list the words were recorded at a constant intensity. Preceding each word is the carrier phrase, "Say the word." Recorded on each of the six records is a 1000 cps tone for calibrating purposes. Both the calibration tone and the carrier phrase are recorded at a level 10 decibels above that of the test words. The point where a normal listener can understand two words out of ten, to where he can understand eight words out of ten, is encompassed within the narrow intensity range of approximately 8 decibels. This steepness of function makes for easy detection of threshold.

C.I.D. Auditory Test W-2 consists of the thirty-six spondaic words of Test W-1 with lists A, B, C, D, E, F. In each list are twelve groups of three words, each group being successively weaker by 3 decibels. The attenuation is such as to afford an average decrease of 1 decibel for each successive word. A 1000 cps calibration tone is provided, and each

* Reprinted here, by permission, from I. J. Hirsh: Development of material for speech audiometry. J. Speech & Hearing Disorders 17: 321-337, Copyright 1952; and The Measurements of Hearing. New York, McGraw-Hill Company, Inc., Copyright 1952.

word is presented after the carrier phrase. The words at the start of each list are recorded at the same level as the calibration tone. The intensity of the carrier phrase decreases, from the ninth word on down, but remains 6 decibels above the test words.

TABLE 2. Words Used for Auditory Tests W-1 and W-2 (Central Institute for the Deaf, St. Louis, Missouri).*

1. airplane	13. greyhound	25. padlock
2. armchair	14. hardware	26. pancake
3. baseball	15. headlight	27. playground
4. birthday	16. horseshoe	28. railroad
5. cowboy	17. hotdog	29. schoolboy
6. daybreak	18. hothouse	30. sidewalk
7. doormat	19. iceberg	31. stairway
8. drawbridge	20. inkwell	32. sunset
9. duckpond	21. mousetrap	33. toothbrush
10. eardrum	22. mushroom	34. whitewash
11. farewell	23. northwest	35. woodwork
12. grandson	24. oatmeal	36. workshop

* These tests are now available on 12-inch phonograph records at either 33⅓ or 78 rpm from Technisonic Laboratories, 1201 South Brentwood Blvd., Brentwood, Missouri.

There is far less standardization of speech audiometry than there is of pure tone audiometry. The wide variations in test equipment and test environment make it essential that an examiner be careful in establishing his normal reference level. Some larger centers make their own disc or tape recordings for test purposes. More often, use is made of the C.I.D. records. We shall consider Auditory Test W-1. Since the words are recorded at a constant intensity, departure can be made from the fixed pattern required in the W-2 test records of descending intensity. The W-1 test can thus be more exploratory and flexible. A threshold study may be lengthened or shortened, while the manner of presentation can be altered to suit the special demands which arise in testing the very young, the aged, the mentally retarded, and language-handicapped individuals.

Phonetically Balanced Words

C.I.D. Auditory Test W-22 contains four basic lists of 50 words each (Table 3). These one-syllable words are all familiar and the lists meet the criteria of phonetic balance, in that the distribution of speech sounds in them approximates a similar distribution in general conversation. Each of the four lists has been prepared in six variations of the word order. The carrier phrase, "You will say", prefaces each word. A 1000 cps calibration tone is included on each disc and approximates the intensity of the carrier phrase and the test words.

Calibration

An essential beginning in accurate hearing measurement is to calibrate one's equipment so that the zero attenuator setting represents the normal threshold of hearing for speech in the context of the particular room, recording, and equipment with which the patient is tested. Calibration should be done with ten or twelve young adults. Care should be exercised to use individuals who are shown by history and examination to have been free of otic disease, and who demonstrate normal hearing for pure tones. With the attenuator dial set at zero, adjust the gain of the amplifier until the point is reached where 50 per cent of the W-1 words are correctly repeated. Then place the stylus on the calibration tone and note the V-U meter reading. This procedure is repeated for each of the normals, and the mean is then determined and noted for reference. Subsequent speech audiometry should include a calibration reference check prior to testing.

TABLE 3. Alphabetical Lists of PB Words Used in Auditory Test W-22.*

List 1	List 2	List 3	List 4
1. ace	1. ail	1. add	1. aid
2. ache	2. air	2. aim	2. all
3. an	3. and	3. are	3. am
4. as	4. been	4. ate	4. arm
5. bathe	5. by	5. bill	5. art
6. bells	6. cap	6. book	6. at
7. carve	7. cars	7. camp	7. bee
8. chew	8. chest	8. chair	8. bread
9. could	9. die	9. cute	9. can
10. dad	10. does	10. do	10. chin
11. day	11. dumb	11. done	11. clothes
12. deaf	12. ease	12. dull	12. cook
13. earn	13. eat	13. ears	13. darn
14. east	14. else	14. end	14. dolls
15. felt	15. flat	15. farm	15. dust
16. give	16. gave	16. glove	16. ear
17. high	17. ham	17. hand	17. eyes
18. him	18. hit	18. have	18. few
19. hunt	19. hurt	19. he	19. go
20. isle	20. ice	20. if	20. hang
21. it	21. ill	21. is	21. his
22. jam	22. jaw	22. jar	22. in
23. knees	23. key	23. king	23. jump
24. law	24. knee	24. knit	24. leave
25. low	25. live	25. lie	25. men
26. me	26. move	26. may	26. my
27. mew	27. new	27. nest	27. near
28. none	28. now	28. no	28. net
29. not	29. oak	29. oil	29. nuts
30. or	30. odd	30. on	30. of
31. owl	31. off	31. out	31. ought
32. poor	32. one	32. owes	32. our
33. ran	33. own	33. pie	33. pale
34. see	34. pew	34. raw	34. save
35. she	35. rooms	35. say	35. shoe
36. skin	36. send	36. shove	36. so
37. stove	37. show	37. smooth	37. stiff
38. them	38. smart	38. start	38. tea
39. there	39. star	39. tan	39. tin
40. thing	40. tear	40. ten	40. than
41. toe	41. that	41. this	41. they
42. true	42. then	42. three	42. through
43. twins	43. thin	43. though	43. toy
44. up	44. too	44. tie	44. where
45. us	45. tree	45. use	45. who
46. wet	46. way	46. we	46. why
47. what	47. well	47. west	47. will
48. wire	48. with	48. when	48. wood
49. yard	49. young	49. wool	49. yes
50. you	50. your	50. year	50. yet

* Technisonic Laboratories have recorded these lists both at 33⅓ rpm and 78 rpm.

Procedure

The hearing loss for speech, or speech reception threshold, can then be determined in a fairly easy manner in most cases. One can begin by estimating the threshold. This used to be done by averaging the pure tone losses for the three "speech" frequencies (500, 1000 and 2000 cps). A better estimate, particularly for an audiogram with a sloping configuration, is to average the two speech frequencies showing the smallest losses. The spondaic words are then presented at a level about 15 decibels above the estimate. The intensity is then reduced in 2, 3, or 5 decibel steps according to the examiner and the unit employed. Threshold is taken to be the lowest level at which fifty per cent of the words are correctly repeated by the patient. Just as the number of test tone presentations in pure tone audiometry is arbitrarily decided, so the number of test words to be given at the various levels is determined by the individual examiner. Threshold exactitude is improved by increasing the number of test words presented, but this should be considered within the practical limits of clinical procedure. Experience will show that it is not necessary to present many words at supraliminal (above threshold) levels. One learns to attenuate so as to arrive at the final threshold in reasonably rapid time. It is probably good practice to utilize six words at the conclusive threshold level.

It is the usual practice to test the better ear first in speech audiometry as in pure tone testing. The need for masking is likewise similar. If there is a difference between the ears of 35 decibels or more in the pure tone frequencies of 500 through 2000 cps, then the better ear should be masked when the poorer ear is being tested with the phones. The nature and amount of the masking noise to be used is still an indeterminate matter. Eighty-five decibels of white noise (re. 0.0002 dynes per square centimeter) can probably be used effectively. Of course, if the speech reception threshold is obtained in the free field then one is testing what is essentially the hearing of the better ear.

The discrimination score is measured with the W-22 word lists both by phones and in the free field. As stated earlier there are fifty words to a list. If all the words are correctly repeated the score is 100 per cent while failure to understand three words results in a loss of six per cent or a score of 94 per cent. The discrimination *score* reflects the number of words correctly heard. Discrimination *loss* is expressed as the percentage of PB words not correctly heard. If ten words are missed then the discrimination loss is 20 per cent. To avoid confusion, *loss* or *score* should be carefully identified.

To obtain the discrimination score the PB words are presented at a level which is well above threshold. What is desired is a measure of the ability of the ear to understand relatively difficult material when it is not limited by the dimensions of its hearing loss for speech. Discrimination testing generally follows the determination of the speech reception threshold for spondaic words. To obtain the maximum PB score the words should be delivered at least 40 decibels above the speech reception threshold. If there is no tolerance difficulty, the test might be given at an even higher intensity level. One complete list of 50 words must be used in order to obtain meaningful results. The discrimination score is simply the number of words heard correctly multiplied by two. Extending the test to a second list of 50 words might result in a more accurate finding.

If the speech audiometer has been calibrated with the W-1 records it becomes necessary to consider that the W-1 calibration tone is 10 decibels above the spondee test words, while the W-22 calibration tone is at about the same level as the PB test words. After adjusting the W-22 calibration tone to the meter reference level, raising the attenuator dial 30 decibels above the speech reception threshold level will yield the desired 40 decibel increase. Sometimes it is valuable to make a detailed exploration of discrimination in the manner of the articulation function. This can be done by obtaining PB scores at successively higher intensity levels (10, 20, 30, 40 decibels, etc.) above the spondaic word threshold. The discrimination score will improve as the intensity is raised until it reaches its maximum. Then, depending on the auditory lesion, as the intensity is raised above the PB maximum level, the discrimination score will either maintain itself or become poorer.

How an individual will react to a stated degree of hearing loss is of course highly unpredictable. One person may find a mild loss to be of catastrophic proportions; another may regard a far greater loss as scarcely handicapping. Determining a therapeutic or rehabilitative program on the basis of audiometric results is very risky unless considered in the broader context of the patient's feelings and his social and economic needs and aspirations. An identical loss might be more devastating to an individual who lived and worked in an area of sophisticated language demands than to another person whose environment encompassed limited language needs. The psychological implications of hearing defects can vary from realistic acceptance of a severe loss to exaggerating a negligible loss to the extent that it serves as an excuse for withdrawing from life's demands.

Examples of Hearing Losses

Figures 14 through 28 depict possible speech test findings for various audiometric contours. These are intended to be neither comprehensive nor definitive but are fairly representative. As stated above, the speech reception threshold can be predicted with fairly good accuracy by averaging the two smallest pure tone losses for the frequencies 500, 1000 and 2000 cps.

At present, prediction of the discrimination score on the basis of air and bone conduction thresholds is best not attempted. Individual variations in pathology, intelligence, desire to hear, ability to synthesize, and many other factors make it essential that the discrimination score be obtained by presenting a standard list of 50 words in a good test environment. Even then the discrimination score will be partly dependent on such external factors as the physical dimensions of the test equipment, whether the material is presented recorded or by live voice, and the vocal apparatus of the speaker.

Fig. 14 represents what is perhaps the most straightforward type of deafness with regard to pure tone-speech test relationships. This is true not only of the speech reception score but can even include the discrimination score. Other than for the external variations just mentioned one may reasonably expect a good discrimination score with conductive deafness.

Fig. 15 represents a mixed deafness, in which bone conduction thresholds are normal for 250 and 500 cps. The maximum discrimination *score* of 92 percent (identical with the notation of 8 per cent *loss*) indicates very little difficulty in understanding speech material which is presented at sufficiently high intensity levels. The mixed deafness pattern of Fig. 16, with near normal bone conduction at 250 cps, has resulted in a discrimination score of 76 per cent. In addition to the quantitative aspects of his hearing loss, as considered by the extent of his departure from the normal threshold of hearing, this individual will encounter a moderate amount of difficulty in understanding difficult speech

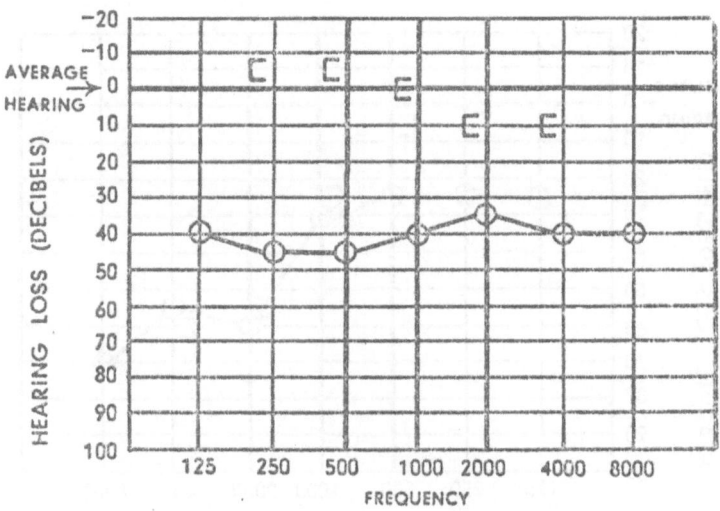

| | SPEECH RECEPTION THRESHOLD (db) | SPEECH DISCRIMINATION LOSS | | | PURE TONES | |
| | | LEVEL (db) | | % LOSS | AVERAGE LOSS 500-2000 (db) | % LOSS (AMA) |
		NOISE	PB s			
BINAURAL						
RIGHT	40			4	40	
LEFT						

Fig. 14—Right conductive deafness.

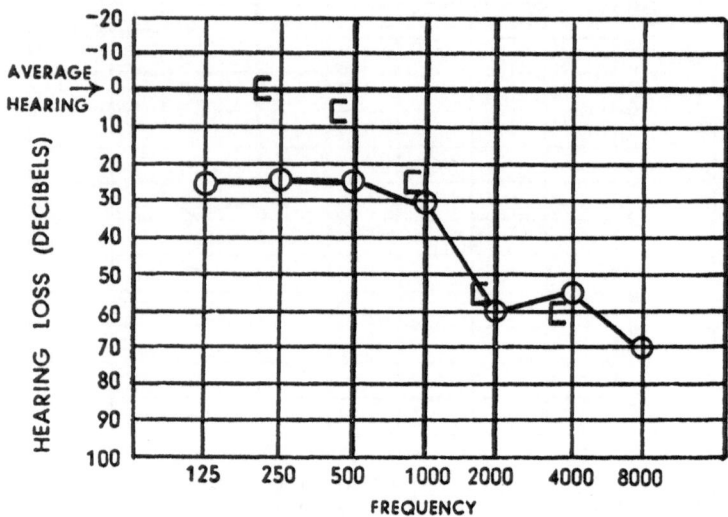

| | SPEECH RECEPTION THRESHOLD (db) | SPEECH DISCRIMINATION LOSS | | | PURE TONES | |
| | | LEVEL (db) | | % LOSS | AVERAGE LOSS ·500-2000 (db) | % LOSS (AMA) |
		NOISE	PB s			
BINAURAL						
RIGHT	32			8	38	
LEFT						

Fig. 15—Right mixed deafness.

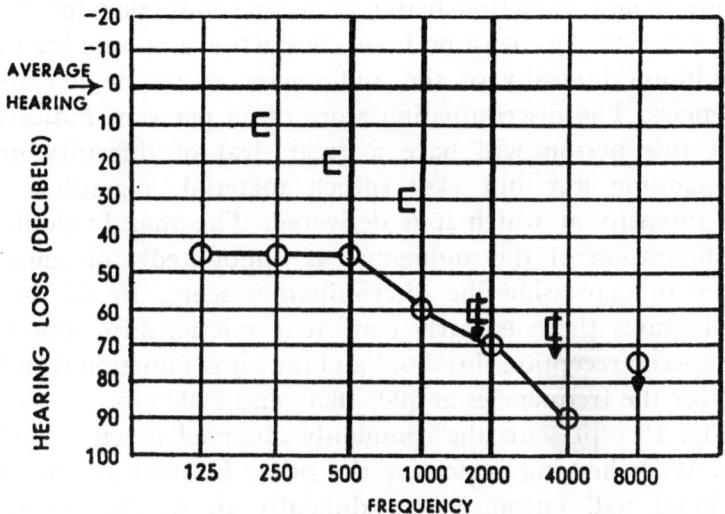

Fig. 16—Right mixed deafness.

	SPEECH RECEPTION THRESHOLD (db)	SPEECH DISCRIMINATION LOSS			PURE TONES	
		LEVEL (db)		% LOSS	AVERAGE LOSS 500-2000 (db)	% LOSS (AMA)
		NOISE	PB s			
BINAURAL						
RIGHT	60			24	58	
LEFT						

material even though it is delivered at high intensities. The audiogram of Fig. 17, also considered in the mixed category, shows bone conduction better than air conduction for 250, 500 and 1000 cps, with no bone conduction response for the maximum intensity of the audiometer at the higher frequencies. The discrimination score of 38 per cent indicates that this person will have a great deal of difficulty understanding any but easy speech material, regardless of the intensity at which it is delivered. The sharply sloping configuration of the audiogram is undoubtedly of importance in depressing the discrimination score. In all three audiograms there is fairly consistent relationship between the speech reception threshold and the air conduction threshold for the frequencies at 500, 1000, and 2000 cps.

Fig. 18 represents the commonly observed notch at 4000 cps. With hearing intact for the other frequencies the individual will encounter no difficulty in hearing or understanding normal speech. The same condition would probably obtain were the hearing defective at 8000 cps. in addition to 4000 cps. In Fig. 19 the perceptive lesion is seen at 2000, 4000 and 8000 cps, with hearing intact for frequencies below 2000 cps. This individual will exhibit little difficulty in responding to speech in our circumscribed test situation. Even the loss illustrated in Fig. 20, with hearing normal only for 125, 250, and 500 cps, will result in only minor difficulty in the speech test situation. Figs. 19 and 20 consider cases of perceptive deafness of a significant degree as measured by pure tone audiometry, but which appear to be within normal limits when examined by our methods of speech audiometry. The explanation lies in the fact that hearing for speech is so closely related to pure tone hearing in the so-called speech frequencies of 500, 1000, and 2000 cps, particularly in the best two of these three frequencies. Hearing losses of the type described in Figs. 19 and 20 will

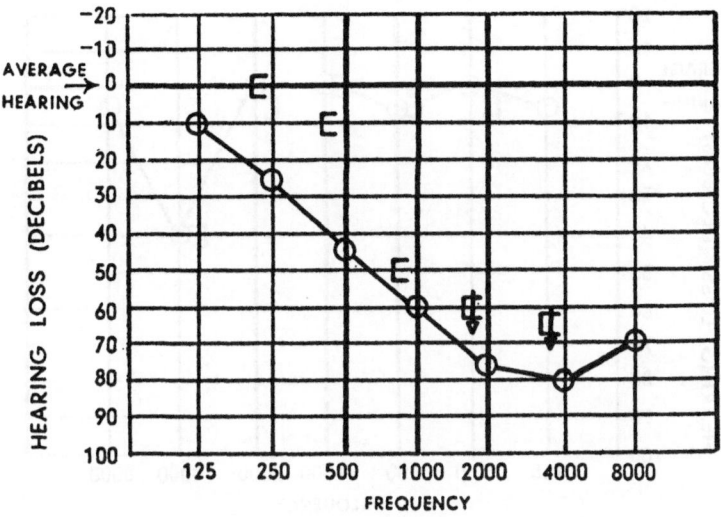

	SPEECH RECEPTION THRESHOLD (db)	SPEECH DISCRIMINATION LOSS			PURE TONES	
		LEVEL (db)		% LOSS	AVERAGE LOSS 500-2000 (db)	% LOSS (AMA)
		NOISE	PB s			
BINAURAL						
RIGHT	60			62	60	
LEFT						

Fig. 17—Right mixed deafness, predominantly perceptive.

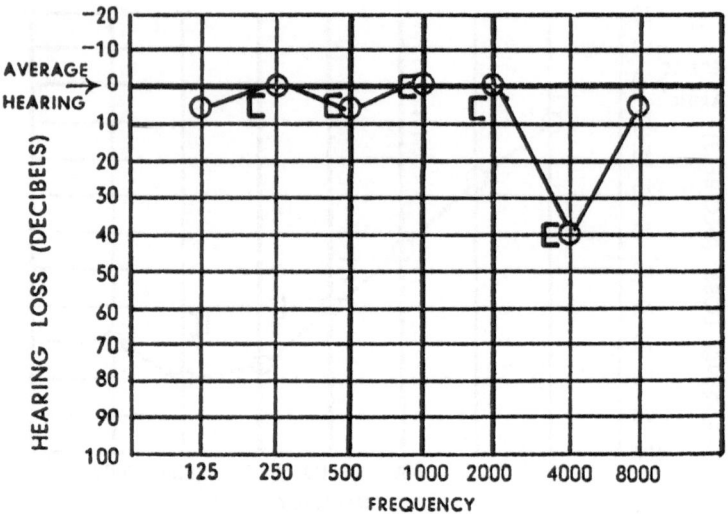

| | SPEECH RECEPTION THRESHOLD (db) | SPEECH DISCRIMINATION LOSS | | | PURE TONES | |
| | | LEVEL (db) | | % LOSS | AVERAGE LOSS 500-2000 (db) | % LOSS (AMA) |
		NOISE	PB s			
BINAURAL						
RIGHT	0			0	2	
LEFT						

Fig. 18—Right perceptive deafness at 4000 cps.

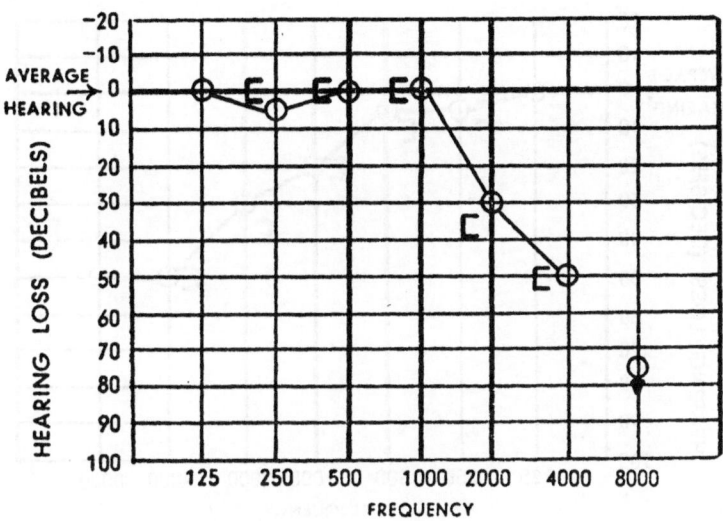

| | SPEECH RECEPTION THRESHOLD (db) | SPEECH DISCRIMINATION LOSS | | | PURE TONES | |
| | | LEVEL (db) | | % LOSS | AVERAGE LOSS 500-2000 (db) | % LOSS (AMA) |
		NOISE	PB s			
BINAURAL						
RIGHT	3			6	10	
LEFT						

Fig. 19—Right perceptive deafness, upper frequencies.

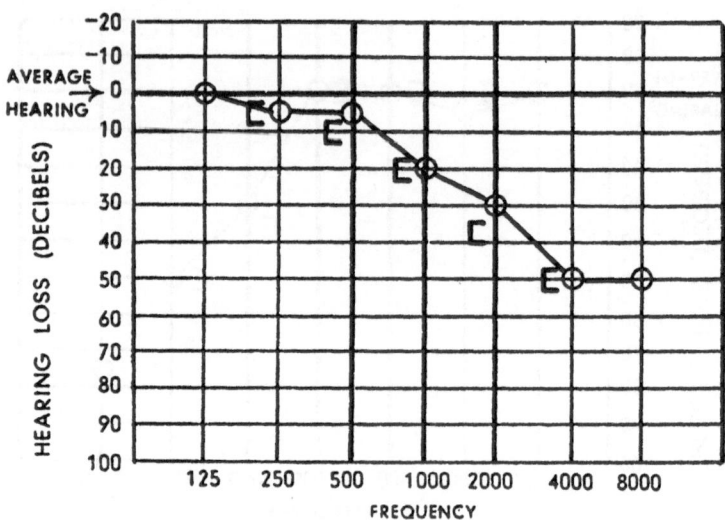

| | SPEECH RECEPTION THRESHOLD (db) | SPEECH DISCRIMINATION LOSS | | | PURE TONES | |
| | | LEVEL (db) | | % LOSS | AVERAGE LOSS 500-2000 (db) | % LOSS (AMA) |
		NOISE	PB s			
BINAURAL						
RIGHT	*14*			*10*	*18*	
LEFT						

Fig. 20—Right perceptive deafness, involving the speech frequencies.

thus have near-normal speech reception thresholds. Clinical evidence further reveals that when the speech reception threshold is fairly close to normal (or not greater that approximately 20 decibels) the individual will obtain a good discrimination score when tested at his maximum intensity level. By our usual speech tests these individuals appear to be within normal limits of hearing, yet it is observed that they frequently are handicapped when listening in a noisy environment, in rapidly shifting group conversation, and in other difficult listening situations.

Perceptive losses heretofore considered have been of the typical sloping configuration, with hearing for the low frequencies much better than for the high frequencies. Figs. 21, 22 and 23 demonstrate varying degrees of perceptive deafness in which the audiometric contour is relatively flat. Again there is fairly close interdependence between speech reception threshold and pure tone thresholds, although it appears that as the loss becomes increasingly severe, the speech threshold exceeds the pure tone threshold. The discrimination score of 78 per cent in Fig. 21 is fairly high for a perceptive loss of this degree, and this individual appears to be operating at a high level of acoustic efficiency within his limitations. Fig. 22 represents a severe perceptive loss which would be very handicapping. The loss portrayed in Fig. 23 is extremely severe both for speech reception and for discrimination. The individual poses a very difficult problem in rehabilitation and can expect minimum success, if any, in using a hearing aid.

Figs. 24, 25, and 26 illustrate varying degrees of disability of the pattern usually seen in Ménière's disease. These individuals usually show reduced discrimination, recruitment, and tolerance problems, all of which tend to place them in the less successful group of hearing aid users.

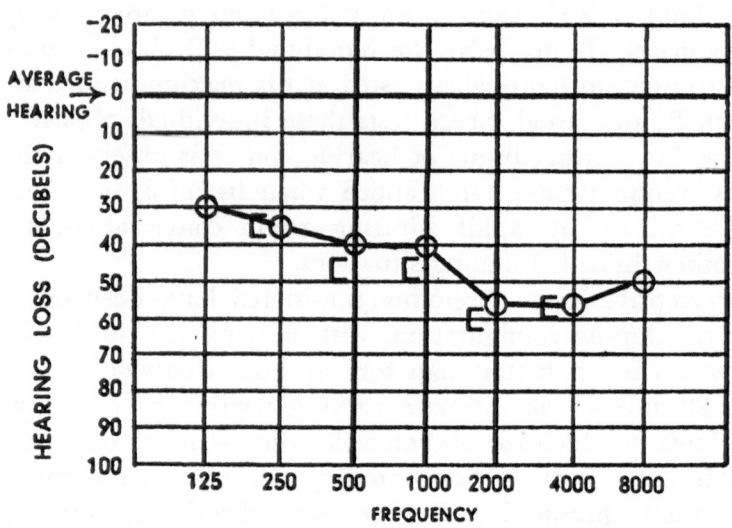

| | SPEECH RECEPTION THRESHOLD (db) | SPEECH DISCRIMINATION LOSS | | | PURE TONES | |
| | | LEVEL (db) | | % LOSS | AVERAGE LOSS 500-2000 (db) | % LOSS (AMA) |
		NOISE	PB s			
BINAURAL						
RIGHT	42			22	45	
LEFT						

Fig. 21—Right perceptive deafness, moderately severe.

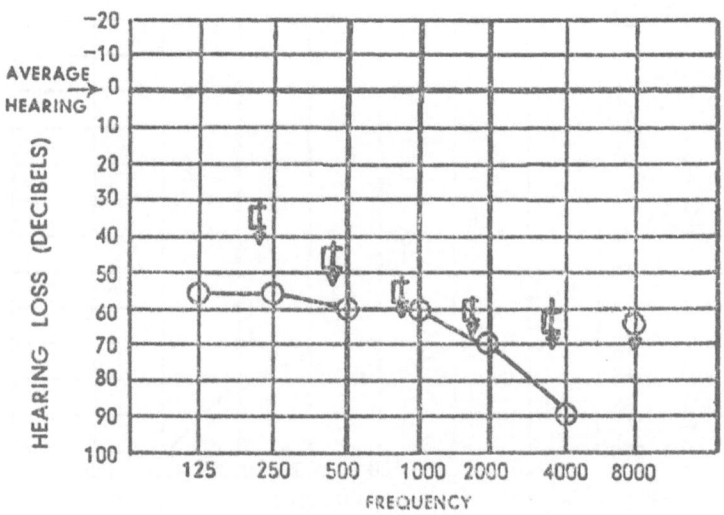

| | SPEECH RECEPTION THRESHOLD (db) | SPEECH DISCRIMINATION LOSS | | | PURE TONES | |
| | | LEVEL (db) | | % LOSS | AVERAGE LOSS 500-2000 (db) | % LOSS (AMA) |
		NOISE	PB s			
BINAURAL						
RIGHT	68			42	63	
LEFT						

Fig. 22—Right perceptive deafness, severe.

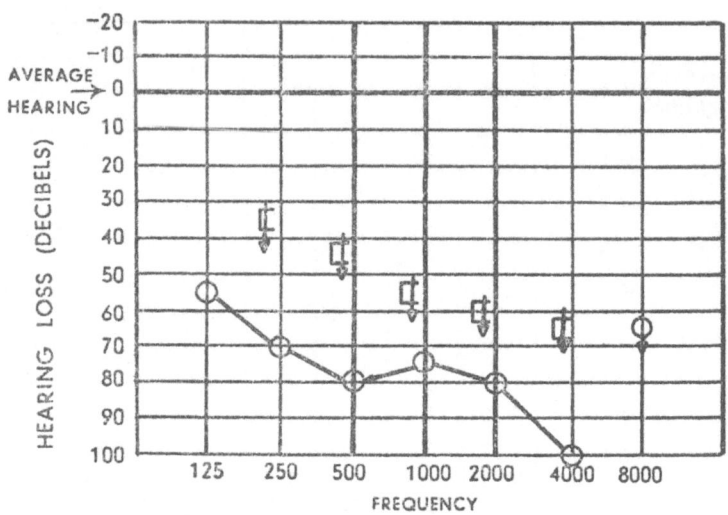

	SPEECH RECEPTION THRESHOLD (db)	SPEECH DISCRIMINATION LOSS			PURE TONES	
		LEVEL (db)		% LOSS	AVERAGE LOSS 500-2000 (db)	% LOSS (AMA)
		NOISE	PB s			
BINAURAL						
RIGHT	86			66	78	
LEFT						

Fig. 23—Right perceptive deafness, very severe.

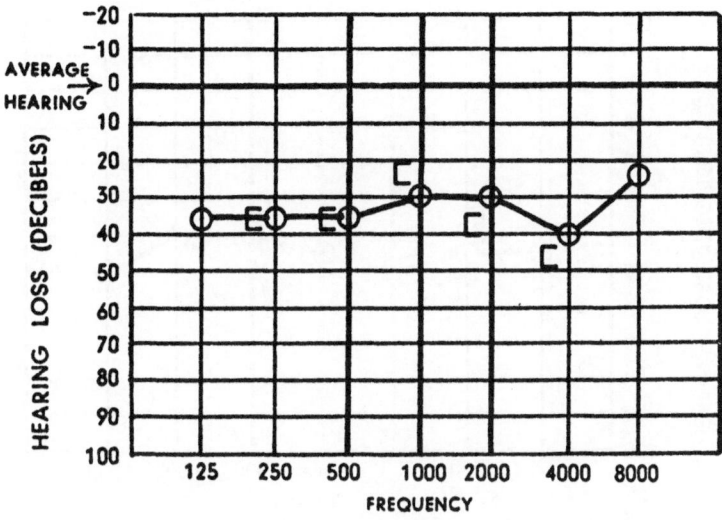

| | SPEECH RECEPTION THRESHOLD (db) | SPEECH DISCRIMINATION LOSS | | | PURE TONES | |
| | | LEVEL (db) | | % LOSS | AVERAGE LOSS 500-2000 (db) | % LOSS (AMA) |
		NOISE	PB s			
BINAURAL						
RIGHT	30			28	32	
LEFT						

Fig. 24—Right perceptive deafness; the clinical diagnosis is Ménière's syndrome.

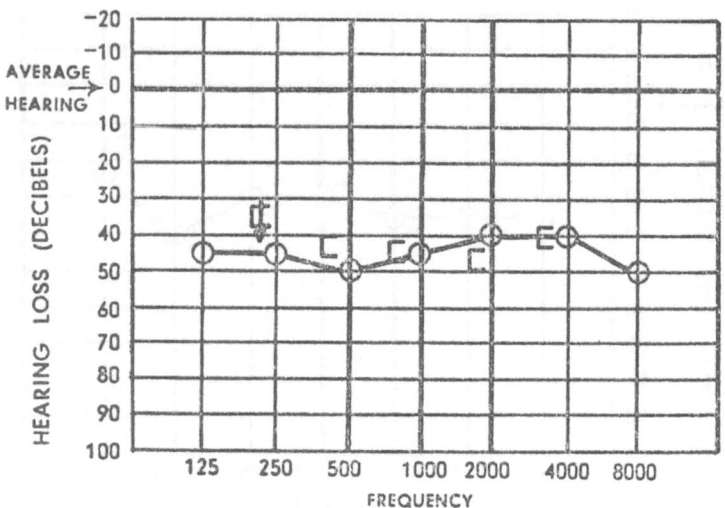

	SPEECH RECEPTION THRESHOLD (db)	SPEECH DISCRIMINATION LOSS			PURE TONES	
		LEVEL (db)		% LOSS	AVERAGE LOSS 500-2000 (db)	% LOSS (AMA)
		NOISE	PB s			
BINAURAL						
RIGHT	52			44	45	
LEFT						

Fig. 25—Right perceptive deafness; the clinical diagnosis is Ménière's syndrome.

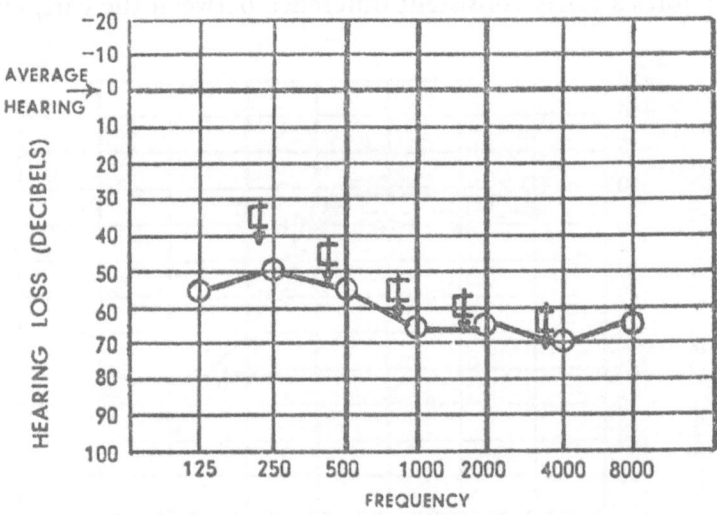

| | SPEECH RECEPTION THRESHOLD (db) | SPEECH DISCRIMINATION LOSS | | | PURE TONES | |
| | | LEVEL (db) | | % LOSS | AVERAGE LOSS 500-2000 (db) | % LOSS (AMA) |
		NOISE	PB s			
BINAURAL						
RIGHT	80			86	62	
LEFT						

Fig. 26—Right perceptive deafness; the clinical diagnosis is Ménière's syndrome.

Fig. 27 and 28 indicate perceptive deafness. Both, the right and left ears, are shown in these audiograms. In Fig. 27 one notes a fairly consistent difference between the ears, and

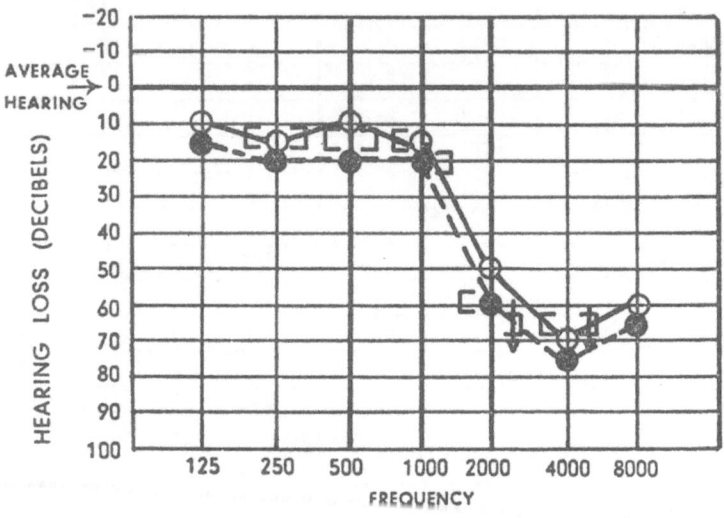

| | SPEECH RECEPTION THRESHOLD (db) | SPEECH DISCRIMINATION LOSS | | | PURE TONES | |
| | | LEVEL (db) | | % LOSS | AVERAGE LOSS 500-2000 (db) | % LOSS (AMA) |
		NOISE	PB s			
BINAURAL						
RIGHT	15			16	25	
LEFT	22			26	33	

Fig. 27—Bilateral perceptive deafness; the differences between the two ears are maintained.

this difference is maintained from the pure tone thresholds to the speech reception thresholds and finally in the discrimination scores. The difference between the ears is 8 decibels for pure tones, 7 decibels for spondee threshold, and 10 per cent for PB discrimination. In Fig.28, however, the right ear has a 37 decibel loss for pure tones with a 28

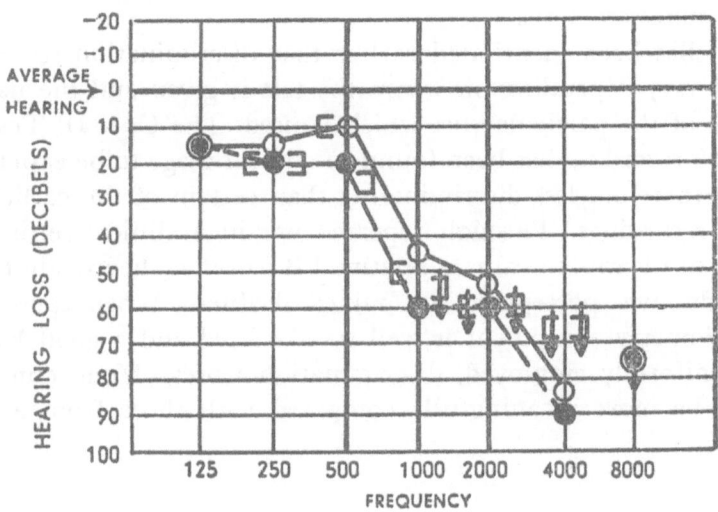

	SPEECH RECEPTION THRESHOLD (db)	SPEECH DISCRIMINATION LOSS			PURE TONES	
		LEVEL (db)		% LOSS	AVERAGE LOSS 500-2000 (db)	% LOSS (AMA)
		NOISE	PB s			
BINAURAL						
RIGHT	28			32	37	
LEFT	36			56	47	

Fig. 28—Bilateral perceptive deafness; the speech reception thresholds are fairly similar but there is considerable difference in discrimination.

decibel loss for speech. The left ear, with a pure tone loss of 47 decibels has a 36 decibel speech threshold. The pattern of consistency vanishes when one observes the discrimination scores which are 68 per cent for the right ear but only 44 per cent for the left. This example indicates how difficult and unreliable it is to predict discrimination scores. These can be accurately obtained only as a result of performing the necessary tests.

It has been mentioned earlier that discrimination scores will vary depending on where the test is given and the nature of the particular list which is used. The C. I. D. Test W-22 recording has been found in clinical usage to be easier, and therefore less discriminating than certain of the earlier PB recordings. Through repeated use in a clinical setting one can learn to evaluate relative PB scores as they relate to conductive, perceptive and mixed deafness. When speech audiometry equipment is well standardized and a good list is uniformly employed, discrimination scores of one clinic can be more meaningfully compared with those from another.

12

HEARING AIDS

For many centuries man has searched for means to over-come hearing impairments. The ear trumpet was one of the earliest devices fashioned to assist the hard of hearing. It has taken many forms in its basic attempt to collect sound waves from a large area and channel them into the external canal. Another early instrument was the speaking tube which is essentially a form of the ear trumpet but designed for direct conversation between two people. An individual with mild perceptive deafness even today might appreciate its lack of distortion and limited amplification. There were also early ingenious bone conduction devices usually consisting of a transmitting rod in contact with the teeth.

The Carbon Hearing Aid

The modern hearing aid has evolved largely from work in the fields of telephone and radio. The earliest electrical hearing aid contained a carbon microphone, battery, cord and magnetic receiver (earphone). These were similar to the telephone in operation. The sound waves impinging on the carbon microphone caused pressure changes between the carbon granules resulting in variations in resistance to the flow of electrical current. The varying current flow, acting

on the magnet of the receiver to strengthen and weaken
its field, resulted in motion of an iron diaphragm placed
near the magnet. The vibrating diaphragm produced sound
waves in the air to complete the cycle begun by the sound
waves which stimulated the carbon diaphragm of the microphone. The small amount of gain developed in this system
necessitated the introduction of a carbon amplifier which
was essentially an additional carbon microphone and magnetic receiver in the circuit. The final product was an instrument of poor quality, relatively low gain, very limited
frequency response, and with various inherent operating
difficulties.

The Vacuum Tube Hearing Aid

Widespread acceptance and use of hearing aids followed
the introduction and development of the vacuum tube instruments. While there have been variations, the basic design employed a crystal microphone, a vacuum tube amplifier, an "A" and a "B" battery, and a magnetic receiver.

The piezoelectric effect is the term used to describe the
conversion of sound pressure vibrations into electrical volt-
ages in the action of the crystal microphone. Sound waves
which strike the diaphragm of the microphone are transmitted to the crystal which is mechanically distorted. This
bending of the crystal results in the production of an electrical charge which corresponds to the initiating sound waves.

The "A" battery of the vacuum tube hearing aid serves
to heat the tube's filament causing electrons to flow from it.
The electrons are drawn to the plate which has a positive
charge placed on it by the "B" battery. The current which
had been generated at the microphone is passed to the grid
of the tube. The alternating negative and positive charge on

the grid acts to manage the electron flow from filament to plate and current flow is thereby controlled.

While some hearing aids have used four, five and even six vacuum tubes, the usual circuit contains three tubes. Since the voltage produced in the crystal microphone is very small, various stages of amplification are provided. In many circuits the first two tubes serve as voltage amplifiers while the third tube assists in the power amplification needed to activate the receiver. An output transformer functions to achieve proper coupling between the final tube and the magnetic receiver.

Batteries

As previously stated the "A" battery current serves to heat the filament of the vacuum tube. A 1.5 volt battery is sufficient for this purpose. The earlier batteries, while called dry cells, actually have a moist mix or electrolyte sealed between the center carbon electrode and the outer zinc electrode. The more recent "B" batteries range from 15 to 30 volts. Some hearing aids use 45 volts by employing two 22.5 volt "B" batteries in series. The "B" battery itself consists of tiny 1.5 volt carbon-zinc cells connected in series to attain the desired voltage. The use of small cells keeps down the overall size of the "B" battery despite its higher voltage.

The voltage of the carbon-zinc "A" battery shows a more or less steady decline with use. This is in contrast to the more recently developed mercury type of "A" battery. Besides certain structural advantages the mercury cell operates in such a manner that the voltage is maintained at an efficient level until it is nearly exhausted, at which time it drops off rather sharply. Apart from the lack of warning this type of decline appears to be more advantageous to a hearing aid user than the steadier voltage drop of the carbon-zinc cells.

Receivers

Earlier vacuum-tube hearing aids employed air conduction receivers of the crystal type. Voltage from the hearing aid amplifier is delivered to the crystal. This results in a bending of the crystal, causing movement of an attached diaphragm. Because of crystal failures in extremes of heat and humidity, the later vacuum-tube aids use magnetic receivers. As described earlier, these depend on a varying current to produce a varying magnetic pull on a diaphragm, with resultant motion of the air in the form of sound waves.

The magnetic receiver is also used as a bone conduction receiver. Here the diaphragm is attached to a case which is positioned on the mastoid bone behind the ear. Movement of the diaphragm causes the case to vibrate against the mastoid bone thereby introducing sound waves into the skull.

The usual method for securing good contact between the bone conduction receiver and the mastoid is to utilize a head band shaped to provide the necessary tension. Bone conduction receivers are used now by only an occasional patient.

Controls

Every hearing aid has a volume control which regulates the gain of the instrument so that the user may hear sounds louder or softer. This is usually obtained by moving a contact along a resistance to allow more or less of the signal to pass.

Some hearing aids have provisions for altering the frequency response so as to obtain a relative enhancement of the high or low frequency bands. The circuit includes combinations of condensors and resistors which may be selected by the wearer. Other aids require internal adjustments by the individual who is fitting the instrument. Generally the wearer effects frequency response changes by means of an external tone control, while the internal controls are of the semi-permanent type not under the patient's command. In some aids variations are obtained by means of receivers which have their own frequency response characteristics and which can be selected to secure desired frequency tilts. In other instruments frequency response is varied by designing a series of models each with a circuit that differs from the others so as to afford a range of possible responses.

Other Components: Cords, Ear-Molds, Garments

Cords. The hearing aid case is made of plastic or metal. It is desirable that it be light in weight, sturdy, and produce a minimum amount of noise when rubbed against the clothing. From the amplifier housed in the case, the current is fed to the receiver by means of the connecting receiver cord. This cord consists of two wires each covered by plastic insulating material. The terminals at each end of the paired wires fit into the jack of the hearing aid and of the receiver.

The terminals vary in size and shape. Some terminals for some hearing aids are uniform, so that they can be inserted into the hearing aid jack or the receiver jack interchangeably. The design of jacks of other aids is such that each terminal will fit into only one jack and sometimes in only one position. It is important that these "polarized" terminals be inserted exactly as the manufacturer has specified in order to avoid breakage of the terminals or jacks, and in order that the aid will operate properly. Usually, polarized terminals are found in hearing aids whose circuit design demands a certain relationship between the receiver and the audio system.

Ear molds. Another item in the hearing aid assembly is the ear mold, or ear insert, for the air conduction receiver, Fig. 29. It is preferable that the insert be made prior to the hearing aid fitting. The standard insert is made of clear or

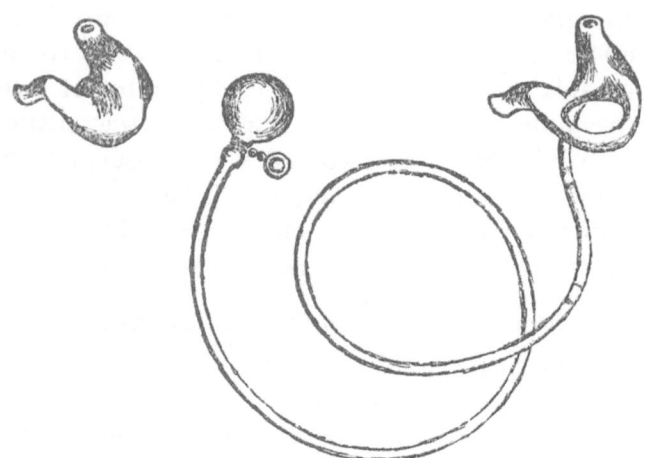

Fig. 29—Ear insert molds: left, standard type; right, invisible contour. The drawings were made from inserts supplied by J. J. Manning, New York City.

tinted acrylic, fabricated from a plastic impression taken of the auricle and external auditory meatus. The adapter of the air conduction receiver snaps into a metal bushing of the insert, and is retained by a ring spring. A good seal between the receiver and insert and between the insert, the auricle, and meatus will eliminate acoustic feedback (squeal) which results when sound escapes from receiver and circles back to the microphone of the hearing aid.

"Invisible" or "skeleton" type ear inserts have been developed and popularized in an attempt to make the wearing of a hearing aid appear to be less conspicuous. A transparent plastic tube extends from the ear insert to the hearing aid receiver which may then be secreted in the woman's hairdo or beneath the man's shirt collar. Since there is an attenuation, particularly for the high frequencies, of sounds which traverse the plastic tube the use of this type of insert is not advisable for many individuals.

A more recent development has been a soft plastic ear

insert. An improved acoustic seal is claimed for this insert
since it tends to adhere to the anatomical contour. In addition it reduces the possibility of traumatic injury to the
ear. There has been a steady increase in the number of
hearing-handicapped younger children who have been ad-
vised to wear hearing aids. Active youngsters wearing an air
conduction receiver may suffer a blow against it and sustain
a laceration of the auricle or canal from a rigid insert. The
recent softer plastic insert may minimize this hazard and be
preferable because of this, provided that it proves satisfactory in other respects.

Garments. Hearing aids are provided with clips by which
they may be attached to a shirt pocket or other appropriate
articles of clothing. Many people prefer to have the instrument out of sight and wear it under the clothing. This is
accomplished by selecting one of several carriers or garments
which are designed for the purpose, Fig. 30. The wearing of
a present-day, small, light hearing aid need not be at all
uncomfortable. A hearing aid which is covered by clothing
operates at somewhat reduced efficiency, particularly for the
high frequencies. In addition it is almost impossible to
avoid the introduction of noise caused by clothing rub.
Nonetheless, most wearers can successfully use a hearing aid
in this manner.

Performance Characteristics

An individual with impaired hearing who turns to a
hearing aid for amelioration of his difficulty does so with the
hope that it will render speech more intelligible to him.
Some people may be more concerned with hearing music,
while to others the ability to hear certain sounds and noises
may be essential to success in job performance. In a large
measure the hearing aid user's satisfaction will rest in a
compromise between his hopes and needs, the actual per-

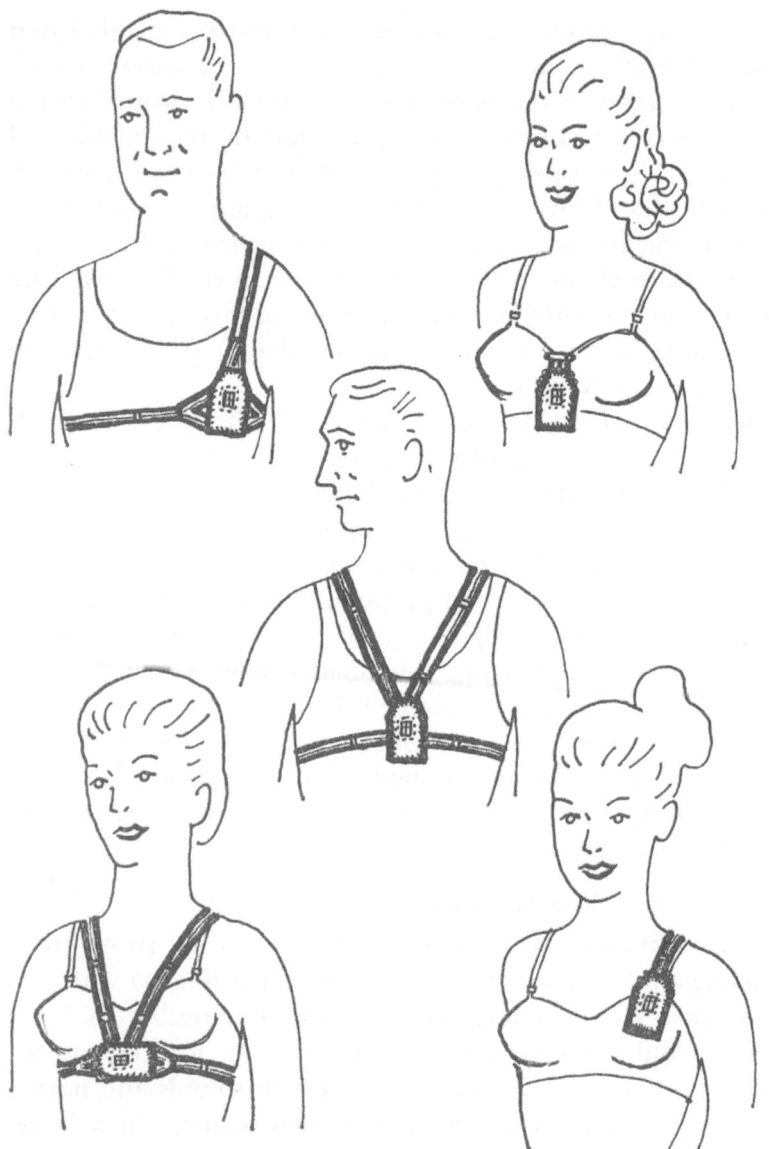

Fig. 30—Garments designed to carry hearing aids, showing several of the styles manufactured by Hechler Brothers, Inc., Long Island City, New York.

formance and limitation of the hearing aid, and the nature of his deafness.

Recent years have witnessed a lively interest in the manufacture of high-fidelity amplifying systems. A system of sound reproduction having a uniform frequency response and which also is linear with respect to intensity must of necessity be both bulky and cumbersome. Hearing aid performance does not even approximate that of high-fidelity audio amplifying systems. While improvements in design will continue, it is quite reasonable to expect limitations and to accept compromises in a small wearable hearing aid.

Frequency Range. The normal young adult can hear sounds within the approximate range of 20 cps to 20,000 cps. This range can be narrowed and still encompass the requirements for a faithful reproduction of orchestral music. For understanding speech, the frequency range may be further restricted since an audio system need not extend beyond 200 cps to 6000 cps., in order to deliver excellent speech intelligibility. While there is considerable variation in the frequency range of the many different hearing aids now available and in use, few if any have a response in excess of 100 cps to 6000 cps. These figures must be considered in terms of the amplification which is produced at the various frequencies. The effectiveness of the frequency range is dependent on there being sufficient amplification available so that the reproduced frequencies may be delivered at a useful level to the hearing aid wearer.

Gain. The primary function of a hearing aid is amplification of sound. An important measure of this characteristic is termed acoustic gain which is taken to be the difference in sound pressure between the output level at the receiver and the input level at the microphone. There is a wide span in the amount of gain provided by the various hearing aids, ranging from approximately 40 to 80 decibels for a 1000 cps signal. Depending on this measure, hearing aids are frequently spoken of as being in the "low-gain," "medium-gain," or "high-gain" categories.

While the gain classifications are usually clinical estimates, the actual acoustic gain can be measured in the laboratory. This is done by placing the hearing aid receiver on an artificial ear. This provides for coupling of the receiver to a 2cc. cavity which simulates the external auditory meatus with ear insert in place. A very sensitive microphone in the artificial ear, together with an associated amplifier network and meter, is used to measure the sound pressure generated at the receiver of the hearing aid being examined. The acoustic gain can be determined by applying a sound pressure of known value to the microphone of the hearing aid while the volume control is turned to maximum gain setting.

Frequency Response Curve. The frequency range and the acoustic gain of a hearing aid are related factors. Determining the acoustic gain at each frequency establishes the frequency response characteristics of a hearing aid. When there is equal gain for each frequency an instrument is considered to have a "flat" frequency response. A "peaked" response characteristic obtains when the amplification at one or two frequencies markedly exceeds the others. Peaking, to a greater or lesser degree, is characteristic of hearing aid frequency response curves. Generally the gain for the mid-frequencies is greater than for the low and high frequency regions. The gain for a particular frequency should be at least 30 to 35 decibels if it is to contribute significantly to speech signal intelligibility.

Maximum Power Output. While acoustic gain and maximum power output of a hearing aid are related to a user's needs, it should be recognized that they are two separate characteristics of an instrument. The gain of a hearing aid describes its ability to amplify sounds, while the maximum output level is the ceiling beyond which the instrument will not deliver regardless of its gain rating. Maximum power output can be determined in the laboratory with the use of an artificial ear. It is measured in decibels (re. 0.0002 dynes per cm²) and is obtained by increasing the level of sound into the microphone until no further increase in output from the receiver can be developed. Variations in the maximum power output among different makes and models of hearing aids range from approximately 110 to 140 decibels for a 1000 cps signal. This cut-off characteristic of a hearing aid is important in connection with the wearer's tolerance for loud sounds.

Distortion. As has been indicated, considerations of size and wearability have resulted in compromises in hearing aid design. This has meant a considerable departure from high-fidelity characteristics. It is not necessary to have identical gain at each frequency since a normal ear cannot detect small deviations from "flat" amplification. When there is a considerable amount of unequal gain for the various frequencies, the quality of reproduction is affected and is termed *frequency distortion.* Pronounced peaks in the frequency response curve are undesirable since they impart a "tinny" quality, may mask adjacent frequencies, and adversely affect tolerability.

The maximum acoustic output of hearing aids is limited. When this limiting level is reached, any further signal increase results in "clipping" of the peaks of the sound pressure. This overloading may interfere with the quality and intelligibility of reproduced speech. This characteristic is termed *amplitude distortion* and is more serious when the low frequencies are involved. As a result of the clipping new tones are produced which were not present in the original signal. These extraneous tones or harmonics constitute a percentage of the total sound output which marks the extent of the amplitude or harmonic distortion.

One advantage of peak clipping is that a maximum output ceiling is imposed on the hearing aid, acting to prevent the production of intensities which might be painful to the user. Compression amplification, another method used to limit output, has theoretical advantages over peak clipping. Modified forms of compression have been tried in hearing aids. While the results have been equivocal, the method offers promise for individuals who need considerable gain, yet have poor tolerance for loud sounds.

Transistor Development

The advent of the transistor has been widely heralded. This electronic device, which was first described in 1948, is considered to be of tremendous scientific and social importance. Some of its potentialities have already been realized while further advances seem assured. It is expected that transistor development will be most startling and fruitful when it is applied in areas in which certain inherent limitations of the vacuum tube may be overcome. Vacuum tubes are relatively short-lived and require considerable power much of which is dissipated in the form of heat. The problem of heat becomes critical when large numbers of vacuum tubes must be used in a small area. Compared to the vacuum tube the transistor is more durable, has a much longer life, and is appreciably smaller. Of major importance is the tremendous reduction in the transistor's power requirements and the elimination of the problems of high temperatures.

Semi-Conductors. Electric current is considered to be a flow of electrons. This can occur in the space of a vacuum tube or in solid matter. The transistor developed out of mastery of current flow in solids known as semi-conductors. Germanium, silicon, and galena crystals are examples of these materials whose properties place them between the good conductors of current such as aluminum or copper, and the insulators or poor conductors of current such as glass or rubber.

In the early days of radio an electrode in the form of a thin wire (cat's whisker) was placed in contact with the surface of a crystalline semi-conductor. This was the crystal detector which acted to pass one half of each cycle of an alternating current thereby converting it into a direct current. The crystal detector soon gave way to the vacuum tube which had the additional capability of amplification.

Work in radar and ultrahigh-frequency transmission during World War II revealed certain deficiencies in vacuum tube operation. Research was redirected to semi-conductors with particular attention to germanium. The result was the transistor, a crystalline semi-conductor able to amplify voltage and power. The concept of current flow as the movement of free electrons from one atom to another obtains for the transistor's germanium crystal. In addition, passage of current in the crystal is further explained on the basis of the movement of "holes" which represent sites in the transistor's crystal structure from which normally present electrons have moved.

Germanium Crystal Production

While transistors can be made with other crystalline semi-conductors, germanium is the commonly used substance. In America it is obtained as a by-product of zinc smelting. Extreme care is given to the purification of the germanium when fabricated into ingot form. Since there is little conductivity in the pure crystalline form, impurities are then added in a highly controlled manner. N-type germanium is produced by the addition of impurities which impart an excess of electrons to the crystal. P-type germanium contains impurities which create a shortage of electrons or the existence of holes or positive charges which move in the direction opposite to that of free electrons. Both types of germanium act as semi-conductors.

Types of Transistors

The *point-contact* transistor is made by placing two thin wires (cat's whiskers) in contact with a germanium crystal. These electrodes are termed emitter and collector while the area where contact is made is the third electrode or base.

The *junction* transistor has been developed more recently. It contains layers of n-type and p-type germanium in either p-n-p or n-p-n assembly, with connections to the layers acting as emitter, collector, and base. The p-n-p junction transistor is the type most frequently used in hearing aid amplification. Depending on which of the two types is used, the flow of either the holes or electrons is controlled by the input signal. In the p-n-p type the greater power of the collector circuit is controlled by an applied signal to the base-emitter circuit.

Transistor Hearing Aids

Since the transistor does not have a filament, an "A" battery to boil off electrons is no longer necessary. A few small 1.25 volt cells meet all the demands of hearing aid use. As a consequence, the transistor hearing aid can be made smaller and less heavy than a comparable vacuum tube instrument; and because of the reduced need of replacing batteries it is much less expensive to operate. This is somewhat counterbalanced by the generally higher initial cost of the transistor type.

A 1.25 volt mercury battery is commonly used in transistor hearing aids, while some others employ the carbon-zinc type. Depending on the particular instrument the number of cells used varies from one to five, or from 1.25 to 6.25 volts. While most of the current models employ three transistors the range is from two to five. There has been improvement in the durability and the reliability of the junction transistors, which together with their longer life should be reflected in greater economy for the user. Another favorable aspect of transistors is their freedom from the ping-like noise of vacuum tube microphonics.

The vacuum tube hearing aid is an instrument of high impedance, high voltage and low current. The transistor hearing aid is a device with low impedance, low voltage and relatively higher current. One result of these differences is that transistor instruments use magnetic microphones which are not as susceptible to the effects of extremes of temperature and humidity as the crystal microphones used in almost all vacuum tube hearing aids. Magnetic receivers are employed in both transistor and vacuum tube hearing aids.

It is difficult to translate the performance characteristics of a hearing aid into a judgment as to whether its tone quality is pleasing or not, since such an estimate is subjective. Experience has indicated that a number of individuals who have used vacuum tube hearing aids have had difficulty in accommodating to the quality of the transistor type. Beginning users of transistor aids have had no greater difficulty in this regard than have beginning users of vacuum tube models.

Transistor and Vacuum Tube Hearing Aids Compared

Gain, maximum power output, frequency response, and degree of distortion are four of the most important characteristics of hearing aids. With regard to the latter two there is probably little difference between transistor and vacuum tube hearing aids. On the other hand, the gain and maximum power output available in a vacuum tube instrument of a given size can now be built into a transistor hearing aid of significantly smaller size. One might then expect this smaller size to be utilized in an extension of gain and power output. That this has not happened is due primarily to the fact that vacuum tube hearing aids have already approached physical and psychophysical limits. These are approximately 80 decibels of acoustic gain and maximum power output of 140 decibels (re. 0.0002 dynes per cm^2). To provide more than 80 decibels of gain would in all likelihood result in acooustic feedback (squeal) that could not be controlled. The sound pressure level of 140 decibels is close to the tolerance threshold for pain.

This analysis would seem to indicate that the advantages of transistor hearing aids lie in the realm of convenience and economy rather than in performance. There is, however, at least one further important difference. The transistor hearing aids are far more versatile and flexible, model for model, then their predecessors. Since a transistor hearing aid can be controlled over a wide range of voltage and current without circuit changes, it has been possible to build instruments which allow for relatively wide alterations in gain and output. A single model can thus be used for disparate cases of hearing loss. At the moment this appears to be an advantage that is more important to the manufacturer than to the wearer, since a person who needs less than the full power available in his instrument is probably carrying a larger hearing aid than his personal needs require. At the same time, the greater flexibility can be advantageous where unusual demands obtain, as in the need for high gain with somewhat reduced power output.

It is well to bear in mind that vacuum tubes have been used and studied for a much longer time than have transistors. The latter are but recently developed and have considerable margin for change and improvement. The vacuum tube had to be "miniaturized" down to hearing aid size. The transistor appeared in its original form in a good size-relationship to hearing aids and still speaks of promising things to come.

Hearing Aid Selection

There has been a good deal of discussion concerning the method of helping the hard of hearing patient select a hearing aid which will furnish him optimum acoustic assistance. Some examiners consider the fitting process to be one of careful measurement while to others it is simply a matter of general guidance. Based on laboratory investigation and clinical experience there have emerged certain principles. What is given here is an outline of techniques and procedures which have proven to be of considerable value in hearing aid selection. The use of a form like that shown in Fig. 31 is helpful.

Deciding Need For A Hearing Aid

Since the primary function of a hearing aid is amplification of speech, its use is reserved for individuals with reduced ability to hear speech. The use of a hearing aid generally is recommended when there is an average loss of at least 30 decibels in the 500-2000 cps audiometric range for the better ear. Equally important as the determination of this minimum level is the necessity for recognizing individual differences. Some people with a loss of more than 30 decibels can function adequately both in terms of their own needs and the demands of their social and vocational milieu. Others find a milder loss to be seriously handicapping.

HEARING AID SELECTION

Name_____Date_____

Previous Aid			Active Condition		
Make	Unaided				
Model					
Receiver					
Battery					
Tone					
Ear					
Gain					
Speech FF	R L				
PB Score db level FF db level	R L				
Noise-speech ratio					
Dynamic range					
Volume					
Tolerance maximum					
Tolerance comfort					
Opinion					

Selection _____   _____

Comments

Aid Issued _____

Fig. 31—Check list for hearing aid evaluation.

The "ideal" candidate for a hearing aid has a conductive impairment with a loss for pure tones which is flat at approximately 50 or 60 decibels. There is a wide range above and below this level which will respond satisfactorily to the amplification furnished by a hearing aid. When the hearing loss, however, is in the region of 90 decibels, scant assistance only can be expected. Some individuals with such severe impairment find a hearing aid to be of value if for no other reason than that it furnishes an awareness of the presence of speech sounds.

There are some patients whose hearing defects are not over-severe, when measured by the pure tone average for 500-2000 cps, who experience great difficulty as hearing aid wearers. If there exists a reduced tolerance for high intensity sounds together with a markedly poor ability to discriminate the sounds of speech, then the prognosis for successful hearing aid use is poor. Instruction in lip reading is important for these individuals. A hearing aid, however, should not be ruled out without a careful investigation of its possibilities.

A larger group than the one just considered consists of patients who have normal hearing for the pure tones through 1000 cps followed by a sharp falling off in acuity for the successively higher frequencies. These individuals will generally have a normal or near normal speech reception threshold with relatively good discrimination when tested at appropriately high levels. The results of testing thus show a loss for pure tones with fairly intact hearing for speech. These patients will usually complain of trouble when trying to hear in a difficult situation, such as listening in a noisy environment or when trying to attend to the rapidly shifting conversation of a group. It is very unlikely that individuals of this kind would derive much benefit from wearing a hearing aid. The instrument would probably compound their troubles in a difficult listening situation, while they do not need help when the listening is relatively uncomplicated and easy.

Determining Ear To Be Used

The recommendation to wear the hearing aid on the better ear is now much more frequently made than heretofore. This is sound procedure particularly when there is severe bilateral loss. If the loss in the better ear is of a mild degree and the poorer ear is still within a usable range, then the latter can be selected; an example is the case of a 35 decibel loss in one ear with a 50 decibel loss in the other. If the poorer ear were at 70 decibels then the aid should be worn on the better ear, which has the 35 decibel loss, to avoid the likelihood of having approximately equal binaural hearing but still of a handicapping nature. The poorer ear usually is not chosen if it has an average pure tone loss in the 500-2000 cps range which is greater than the corresponding loss in the better ear by 25 or 30 decibels or more. Another consideration is to select the ear with the lesser pure tone air conduction slope in configuration, and one which has the better discrimination.

Sensitivity

The amount of amplification provided by a hearing aid is taken to be a measure of its gain or sensitivity. The greater the degree of a patient's hearing loss the greater must be the gain of his hearing aid. The determination of an instrument's performance in this regard follows the unaided speech audiometry and should be obtained in an acoustically adequate two-room testing suite. The hearing aid is attached to the hearing aid baffle *(See Chapter 3)* immediately behind and just above the patient's chair. The examiner can converse with the patient by using the microphone circuit of the hearing evaluator assembly. As occasion demands he will leave the control room to speak directly to the patient in the sound-treated room and to make the necessary adjustments in the volume and tone control setting of the hearing aid under trial.

The sensitivity of a hearing aid generally is used to determine minimum adequacy of a hearing aid. The examiner uses an ordinary or slightly reduced conversational level while speaking to the patient who now has the hearing aid with the ear insert (preferably custom made) in place. The examiner alters the volume control setting seeking an adjustment which the patient considers to be comfortable for his present listening. The examiner then returns to his equipment and obtains the speech reception threshold. Under these circumstances the patient's aided threshold is usually found to be approximately 35 decibels better than his corresponding unaided speech reception threshold. In presenting the spondaic words used in this measurement, either monitored live voice or recorded material can be used. Generally the use of a tape reproducer or phono player will be found most advantageous. Where improvising is necessary, as in working with children, the use of monitored live voice is preferred.

Testing for sensitivity is used by some examiners as a criterion in determining selection predicated on test score differences which may be established. When this is done it is necessary to set the volume control on the basis of a standard speech input. Recorded continuous speech is introduced, usually at a level 40 decibels above normal threshold, and the volume control of the hearing aid is set for comfort. Differences in aided speech reception threshold are then noted as one proceeds from hearing aid to hearing aid. Differences in sensitivity of 6 decibels or less are not considered to be significant. While it is expected that a hearing aid prove itself satisfactory by furnishing a sufficient amount

of amplification, it is open to question whether differences
between hearing aids on this basis should be used as a factor
in selection. Obtained differences in the aided speech reception threshold are meaningful only if the patient can
set the volume control of the various hearing aids with uniform accuracy at the time he is listening to the running
speech. Not all patients can make consistent settings of the
volume control on the basis of the loudness of perceived
speech.

Discrimination Score

The unaided speech audiometry will have included a test
for discrimination employing a list of 50 PB words presented at a level 40 decibels above the speech reception
threshold. Using the additional PB lists, discrimination
scores are obtained with the various hearing aids in place.
Differences of less than 6 per cent (3 test words) are not
considered significant. The criterion of discrimination is an
important one in hearing aid selection and large differences
between aids should be weighted accordingly. However, one
should not expect the aided discrimination score to surpass
the unaided score. Often the aided discrimination score will
be poorer since the electroacoustic characteristics of a hearing aid are far below the quality of the usual large hearing
evaluator assembly used in obtaining the unaided percentage.

Thus far the hearing aid performance has been assessed
in the relative quiet of a sound-treated room. Were this
testing done in an ordinary noise environment the conditions might be more realistic. However, outside the sound-
treated room the real life noise level is constantly shifting
and controlled measurements from hearing aid to hearing
aid become impossible. A way of meeting this problem is
to introduce a measured noise into the sound-treated room.

Calibrated white noise measured from normal hearing threshold is satisfactory for this purpose. The PB words are presented at a level 40 decibels above the speech reception threshold with an accompanying background of white noise 30 decibels above the speech reception threshold. The discrimination score with noise 10 decibels below the level of the speech signal is obtained unaided and with various hearing aids which are being investigated. This test is usually more rigorous for those persons who have difficulty understanding the PB words in quiet.

Tolerance and Dynamic Range

These factors can be determined in related test sequences. Following the original setting of the volume control for the comfort level the aided speech reception threshold was obtained. The intensity of the speech signal is then increased. The intensity may be raised in 5 or 10 decibel steps until it is 50 decibels above normal threshold. From this point on the intensity is increased cautiously in 2 or 3 decibel increments until the patient reports intolerability or extreme discomfort. This test must be done carefully since a new hearing aid user in particular may become very disconcerted when his tolerance level is reached. Besides the tolerance measure, the test shows the dynamic range of intelligibility from low to high input levels while the volume control is maintained at the comfort setting.

The next step in this procedure is to adjust the volume control of the hearing aid to its maximum setting and repeat the tests as above thus determining the minimum intelligibility and the maximum tolerability of which the instrument and patient are capable. Tolerance thresholds can be determined using connected discourse or white noise. However by employing the spondaic words, it is easy to obtain the desired minimum threshold. In addition, as the intensity is raised, one may note that with an occasional patient the words cease to be intelligible while remaining tolerable. In performing these tests it is not necessary to explore the dynamic or operating range below 10 decibels or above 85 decibels re normal threshold. The upper limit will not be exceeded by a hearing aid at maximum gain setting while the lower level is so soft that speech is almost certain to be masked by ambient noise in all but controlled conditions. It is of course desirable to select a hearing aid with a wide dynamic range and one which gives the least tolerance difficulty.

Quality

Following the unaided speech audiometry the tests are performed completely with each hearing aid. The patient's estimate of the quality of the instrument is then obtained. The procedure is repeated with other hearing aids. In many cases, particularly those of moderate, uncomplicated, conductive deafness, significant differences in the test scores will not develop. The deciding factor may then be the patient's subjective opinion of how each of the instruments sounds to him. A simple rating scale can be set up for judging and scoring the quality of each instrument, or the patient may merely indicate the order of preference for the various hearing aids tested. A related item is whether any of the instruments produce excessive amounts of internal noise.

General Consideration. Among the characteristics which do not readily lend themselves to measurement, the factor of hearing aid size has ceased to be an important one. The use of transistors has led to instruments of considerably reduced size and weight. Since electroacoustic equipment is subject to breakdown, the availability of hearing aid repair service should be considered. Other things being equal, it is preferable to select a hearing aid for which adequate local repair facilities are obtainable by the patient.

Hearing tests and a hearing aid fitting should always be preceded by adequate otological examination. Medical or surgical alleviation of hearing losses offers many patients an amelioration of their impairment with restoration of serviceable hearing. It is to be emphasized again that deafness is the functional impairment symptomatic of organic or psychological disease, or both.

Another otological consideration concerns the meatal insert. Only a physician can evaluate properly contraindications in the use of an ear mold because of some pathological, anatomical, or post-operative limitation.

There is a tendency in some quarters to consider the need for a detailed hearing aid selection procedure as being limited to a small percentage of cases. This is predicated on the belief that most hard of hearing individuals can be benefited equally by any of a fairly large number of good hearing aids. It is probably true that significant test differences will not appear in many of the "easy" cases. However, if an individual with a 40 decibel loss of a conductive nature obtains a hearing aid with 80 decibel gain, then it becomes an example of an "easy" case that has been improperly fitted. Conversely, an individual with severe conductive impairment may select a low gain instrument if left to his own devices. This, too, illustrates how it is very possible for a straightforward case to be poorly treated. A careful process of hearing aid selection or fitting should be performed in all instances of hearing loss of a very mild or severe degree. Thorough fitting is required also whenever there are problems of reduced tolerance thresholds, difficulty in discrimination, and in practically every instance of perceptive deafness.

Hearing aids are imperfect instruments. They are not

adaptable to an exactness of fitting. They do not identify the direction from which sounds emanate. With satisfactory monaural amplification a patient experiences the problems of other people with monaural deafness. Hearing aids do not provide high-fidelity reproduction. It is well to advise patients of the limitations of hearing aids and to strive for their realistic acceptance of the handicaps of deafness and to accept the great potentials for improvement which electro-acoustic amplification provides. Auditory rehabilitation offers additional support in the medical care of the acoustically handicapped.

13_____

VOICE AND SPEECH PRODUCTION

Recognition is the identification of a person or thing already known. We recognize known persons not merely by their physical appearances, but by the way their voices sound to us. In many instances we use only the voice and speech patterns as a means of identification. For example, during a telephone conversation we frequently are able to recognize the speaker by his manner of speaking before he identifies himself by name. The speaker may change his voice by altering the vocal musculature which prevents us from identifying him solely from his speech patterns. By pinching his nose with his fingers while speaking or by placing a handkerchief over the telephone mouthpiece, the speaker changes his normal speech patterns so that recognition of the known voice becomes less likely. These changes are deliberate and voluntary.

The following chapters will describe changes in voice and speech patterns which do not occur voluntarily. Some of these changes are symptomatic types of pathology of the vocal mechanism which generally will occur when there is a disruption of the normal pathways of air set into vibration and perceived as speech.

The primary purposes of respiration are to permit the exchange of oxygen and carbon dioxide and to eliminate water. Speech is considered an overlaid function of recent acquisition. The source of vocal expression is the flow of air from the lungs, with only occasional exceptions (i.e. laryngectomy with esophageal speech). The lungs are situated in the thoracic cavity, the base of which is a horizontal partition, the diaphragm, and the sides of which are made by the ribs and intercostal muscles. The capacity of the thoracic cavity can be made larger or smaller and air can be sucked into or expressed from the lungs through the trachea and larynx by controlling the diaphragm, the intercostal muscles, and other accessory respiratory muscles. During normal phonation air escapes from the lungs; the rate and regularity being controlled by these groups of muscles. A complex structure, tubular in shape, the larynx, is superimposed upon the proximal end of the trachea.

The larynx contains a pair of muscular bands, the true vocal cords, and breath forced out through the rima glottis causes them to vibrate. The expired air, thrown into vibration by variations in the approximation of the tensed vocal cords, is divided into minute puffs which are expelled into the oral and nasal cavities and perceived as sound. The pitch of the voice can be modified by the many alterations of the vocal cords (length, thickness, and tension) . Modifications of voiced sounds (sounds produced by vibrations of the vocal cords) and unvoiced sounds (sounds produced without vibration of the cords) are affected by the tongue, soft palate, hard palate, lips, teeth, and the confining walls of the hypopharynx, pharynx, oropharynx, nasopharynx and nose. The adjustable and flexible combinations formed by these rigid and soft parts and the breath stream produce speech. The chambers of the throat, mouth and nose affect the quality of the phonation. Tonal changes are produced particularly by the alterations of the cavities of the mouth and throat, the nasal cavity being of lesser importance as a resonator.

Vocal Sounds

Voice refers to the basic tone originating in the larynx. The vocal cords, tensed by muscular action and from the stream of air below, vibrate, driving the air into the cavities of the throat, mouth and nose. Here it is selectively amplified, modified and interrupted by the articulators, and emerges from the mouth as speech sounds. Voice is the carrier of what we hear, while speech is the agent of intelligibility. For example, voice can be compared with molten steel, and speech with the many different shapes into which this molten metal is processed.

Vocal sounds have four basic or fundamental characteristics: volume, pitch, quality and rate.

Volume is a measure of the energy produced while speaking. An increase or decrease in the amount of energy will result in similar changes of volume. Volume is deemed adequate when it has sufficient fullness or quality for achieving the demands made upon it by the audience situations and the type of material uttered.

Pitch refers to the position of the voice on a musical scale and is related to the frequency of sound waves. The fundamental sound is determined by the frequency of vibrations of the vocal cords. Pitch consists of two elements: *Key,* the average pitch from which a tone may rise and fall in comfort; *inflection* or *intonation,* the melody patterns produced as the voice rises and falls from one pitch to another. Pitch is deemed adequate if it has appropriate speech melody; proper upward and downward shifts of voice essential to convey shades of meanings and purposes at a level which is suitable to the speaker and to the material spoken.

Quality of tone refers to the pitch and its means of resonance. After a tone is initiated it is reinforced by the walls of the throat, mouth or nose. Quality is deemed acceptable when the flexible walls of the resonators respond promptly and correctly to the demands of the speaker so as to characterize and color the various speech sounds. The reinforcement of tones produces proper shadings and harmony patterns, essential in the production of appropriate sounds. These properly reinforced or resonated tones sound suitable to the listener and are clear enough to be heard above the ambient noise.

Rate of speech refers to the element of time. Rate is deemed acceptable when it adjusts itself to meet the demands or mood of a particular listener or audience; when it is suitable in relative length of individual speech sounds and pauses; and when it has adequate speech rhythm for the material.

Speech Sounds

Speech sounds, phonemes, are classified into three major groups, predicated on the manner in which the expired breath is conditioned by the organs of vocalization: (1) consonants, vowels and diphthongs, (2) voiced or breath sounds and voiceless or breathless sounds, and (3) oral and nasal sounds.

A consonant, voiced or unvoiced, is a speech sound produced by the escaping air being constricted or impeded somewhere in the vocal passages resulting in a friction noise.

A phoneme is considered to be a vowel when the voiced breath is produced with little or no obstruction. It receives its characteristics from the adjustments made in the size of the oral and pharyngeal cavities and by the size of their apertures.

Voiced or breath sounds are those speech sounds produced when the air has been set into vibration by the approximation of the vocal cords so that a murmur is produced.

Unvoiced or breathless sounds are produced when the air, escaping through the glottis, is not set into vibration but is impeded or adjusted in its outward passage so that a slight noise is produced.

Oral sounds are those speech sounds phonated through the throat and mouth; nasal sounds are those sounds produced by directing the vibrated air through the nose.

Consonants

Consonants may be categorized into two principal groups: (1) by the manner of formation, (2) by the site of articulation and whether the air has been set into vibration or no impedance is set up until after the air stream passes through the glottis.

Regarding the manner of formation, consonants can further be classified into four sub-groupings: plosives, fricatives or sibilants, nasals, and glides.

Plosives or stops are so named because the breath is compressed and then suddenly released or exploded (P, B, T, D, K, G).

Fricatives occur when the manner of production results in a constriction of the air which is forced out producing a friction-like noise (F, V, TH, H, R). Certain high frequency fricatives are classified separately as sibilants (S, Z, SH, CH, ZH, as in azure, J).

There are three sounds in the English language which are classified as nasal sounds, so labeled because the air is resonated in the nasal cavity (M, N, NG).

The four sounds in the English language known as glides are the result of gliding movement of the tongue or the lips or both during their production (L, R, W, Y).

By site of articulation consonants can be classified as follows:

1. *Lip* or *bi-labial.* Outgoing breath is impeded or stopped at the lips. (P—unvoiced plosive; B—voiced plosive; M—voiced nasal continuant, breath being emitted in a continuous stream; W—unvoiced frictionless continuant; WH—unvoiced frictionless continuant.)

2. *Lip-teeth* or *labio-dental.* Outgoing breath is impeded by the lower lip being brought up against the upper teeth. (F—unvoiced fricative continuant; V—voiced fricative continuant.)

3. *Tongue-teeth* or *lingua-dental.* Outgoing breath is impeded by the tongue tip being placed against the upper teeth. The tongue may also be placed between the teeth and the air stream is allowed to flow gently over the tongue. (TH—unvoiced fricative continuant; TH—voiced fricative continuant.)

4. *Teeth-ridge* or *lingua-alveolar* (gum ridge). Tip of the tongue approximates against the upper alveolar ridge. (T—unvoiced stopped; D—voiced stopped; N—voiced nasal continuant; L—lateral continuant; S—unvoiced fricative continuant [sibilant]; Z—voiced fricative continuant [sibilant]; R—voiced fricative continuant [semi-vowel]; SH—unvoiced fricative continuant [sibilant]; ZH—voiced fricative continuant [sibilant]; CH—voiced stopped fricative [sibilant]; J—voiced stopped fricative [sibilant].)

5. *Lingua-palatal.* The front of tongue approximates against the hard palate. (Y—unvoiced fricative as in the word "yes".)

6. *Soft palate* or *lingua-velar.* The back of tongue approximates against the soft palate or velum. (K—unvoiced stopped; G—voiced stopped; NG—voiced nasal continuant.)

7. *Glottal.* The glottis is narrowed so that the air passing through it causes friction, but not sufficient to produce voicing. (H—unvoiced fricative continuant).

Vowels

Vowels have two important characteristics: *Resonance* and *absence of audible friction*. Each vowel has its own special resonance. Once the vibrating air stream is emitted through the glottis it undergoes changes of resonance in the mouth or vowel chamber. It is the resonance of a certain part of the chamber only which gives any vowel sound the individual quality which distinguished it from the other vowels.

Vowels can be divided into groups according to the position of the tongue during phonation. They are grouped as front vowels, middle vowels, and back vowels. The position of the lips, such as rounded, unrounded and widely open, unrounded and opened in a narrow slit—also characterize vowel production. Tensity or laxity causes a difference of the walls of the vocal passage thus further influencing vowel production. Length of vowel, (long, half-long, and short) is another determinant of vowel production.

Vowels are classified as follows:

Front vowels. Long E as in the word *see* (tense); short I as in the word *it* (lax); long A as in the words *day, they, April* (tense); short E as in the word *let* (lax); intermediate A as in the word *ask* (lax); short A as in the words *airplane, dare* (tense).

Middle vowels. Long UR as in the word *fur* (tense); middle A as in the word *about* (lax); U as in the word *up* (lax).

Back vowels. Long OO as in the word *moon* (tense); short OO as in the word *foot* (lax); long O as in the word *no* (tense); broad O as in the word *for* (tense); short O as in the word *not* (tense); long A as in the word *garden* (lax).

Diphthongs

A diphthong is a compound sound consisting of the blending of two vowels so heard that there is no sonority between them. Diphthongs occurring in the English language are as follows:

A combination of short E as in the word *let* and short I as in the word *it* forms the sounds of A as in the word *sane*, EY as in the word *they*, and AI as in the word *wait*.

A combination of intermediate A as in the word *ask* and short I as in the word *it* forms the sounds of I as in the word *ice*, AI as in the word *aisle*, EI as in the word *sleight*, Y as in the word *style*, and IE as in the word *pie*.

A combination of long O as in the word *open* and the short OO as in the word *foot* forms the sounds of OU as in the word *bough*, OW as in the word *cow*, and AU as in the word *sauerkraut*.

A combination of the broad O (AW) as in the word *saw* and the short I as in the word *it* forms the sounds of OI as in the word *oil* and OY as in the word *boy*.

A combination of the short I as in the word *it* and middle A as in the word *about* forms the sounds of EA as in the word *idea*, EE as in the word *steer*, IE as in the word *bier*, and the first E as in the word *here*.

A combination of short A as in the word *air* and middle A as in the word *about* forms the sounds of A as in the word *fare*, AI as in the word *airplane*, EA as in the word *pear*, EI as in the word *heir*, and the first E as in the word *there*.

A combination of either short O as in the word *not* or short OO as in the word *foot* and middle A as in the word *about* forms the sounds of OA as in the word *oar*, O as in the word *more*, OO as in the word *floor*, and OU as in the word *pour*.

A combination of broad O (AW) as in the word *saw* and middle A as in the word *about* forms the sounds of OO as in the word *boor*, U as in the word *sure*, and OU as in the word *tour*.

In the production of speech and speech sounds, generally, little or no deviation from the norm occurs when there is no pathology of the vocal mechanism present. However, when some pathology of the mechanism responsible for the normal production of speech and speech sounds appears, an individual demonstrating a malfunction will manifest many voice and speech changes associated with the area of dysfunction. Voice and speech changes which occur because of pathology frequently may be utilized as a means of differential diagnosis of the possible areas of the dysfunction and provide clues to the nature and degree of malfunction.

Pathology Manifested in Voice and Speech

Dysfunction of the oral musculature and their resultant voice and speech manifestations are as follows:

Nasal Passages and Nasopharyngeal Pathologies

(1) Obstruction of the nasal passages, rhinolalia clausa anterior, frequently causes nasality or hyper-nasality. Vowels and semi-vowels are nasalized with the nasal consonants M, N, NG muffled. Often this type of nasalization has been described as a "nasal twang." Examples of this speech deviation are associated with or secondary to deviated septum, turbinal hypertrophy, and chronic allergic rhinitis.

(2) Obstruction of the nasopharyngeal airway, rhinolalia clausa posterior, or negative nasality, frequently produces denasalization of the nasal sounds M, N, NG. A common or frequent example of these substitutions is noted or observed in individuals suffering an acute rhinitis, or an acute allergic rhinitis. Some examples of these aberrations are heard when the word *my* sounds like *by*, the word *no* sounds like *do*, and the word *sing* sounds like *sig*. Contributing causes to this kind of speech are sinusitis, enlarged adenoids, rhinal

polyps (anterior or posterior or both), rhinal foreign bodies (anterior or posterior or both), neoplasms (anterior or posterior or both) and scar formation (depending on location).

Pathology of the Oropharynx

(1)Paralysis of the velum and cleft palate, rhinolalia aperta, frequently produces a speech pattern characterized by marked nasality and absences of the explosive characteristics of K, G, T, D, P, F, V, S, Z, SH, CH. These sounds are seriously weakened.

(2) Harelip or cleft lip may disturb only those sounds involving the upper lip such as P, B, M, U, W. When the upper teeth and gum ridges are also involved, the sounds of voiced and unvoiced TH, F, V, S, Z are produced defectively.

(3) Abnormalities of the dentition, of the maxilla and of the mandible, frequently affect the proper articulation of many speech sounds. Some of these deviants are the S, Z, CH, J, TH, P, B, M, N sounds.

Pathology of the Tongue

Microglossia, macroglossia, paralysis of the tongue, and short or tight frenulum frequently will produce speech deviations ranging from overall defective articulation to broadly defective utterance of S, Z, SH, CH (lisping) and sound substitutions.

Laryngeal Pathology

(1) Congenital anomalies frequently produce a muffled, hoarse abnormal quality.

(2) Paralysis, vocal abuse, chronic laryngitis, and nodules, and neoplasms frequently cause hoarseness, pitch breaking or even aphonia.

(3) Laryngeal disease, pathology, or malfunction caused by thoracic, cervical, metabolic, infectious, systemic or

neurologic diseases as manifested by symptoms of impaired voice, dysphasia and, at times, dysphagia.

Psychological Factors

So-called hysterical aphonia—psychosomatic aphonia, split voice, adolescent voice of the adult, weak voice, etc.

A knowledge of the voice and speech changes manifested by pathology of the vocal mechanism can be used in the examination of patients with voice or speech defects. Similarly, this methodology can also be applied in the diagnosis of individuals alleging a loss of hearing. Speech is the motor manifestation of acoustic function. A loss of hearing will, therefore, manifest itself in many voice and speech deviations.

Elements of the Communicative Process

Speech is a communicative process and speech skills are an outgrowth of speech itself. Speaking and hearing, two elements of the communicative process, are so closely related that a serious impairment in either will frequently result in a breaking down of the entire process. Such disruption of communication will often produce extensive psychological and sociological results.

Language in the infant is learned exclusively through hearing. Although the potential for speech is inborn, language itself is a learned process. When a loss of hearing occurs, an individual frequently develops poor speech habits and acquires speech mannerisms which deviate from the normal speech and voice patterns. The normal hearing ear is the director of phonation, and monitors vocalization and verbalization. A barrier to proper monitoring is raised by deafness; the type, severity and duration of the hearing impairment will be reflected in voice and speech deviations that are trademarks of particular types of deafness. A trained listener can frequently judge the kind of deafness by voice and speech patterns of the individual so handicapped.

Definitions

In the field of speech and hearing, definitions of the terms hard of hearing, deaf and deafened are as follows:

Hard of hearing or *impaired hearing*. An individual is hard of hearing when he has no less than 30 decibels loss nor more than 75 decibels loss of hearing in the better ear after the age at which voice and speech patterns were acquired through the normal channels of hearing.

Deaf. An individual is deaf when he has sustained a complete loss of hearing or the greater part of his hearing (70 to 75 decibels) in the better hearing ear *before* the age at which voice and speech patterns were acquired through the normal channels of hearing.

Deafened. An individual is deafened when he has sustained a complete loss of hearing or the greater part of his hearing (70 to 75 decibels) in the better hearing ear *after* the age at which the voice and speech patterns were acquired or established through the normal channels of hearing.

14

SPEECH DEVIATIONS IN
CONDUCTIVE DEAFNESS

Conductive, impedance deafness is an impairment of hearing due to a defect of the transducing mechanism of the middle ear or a failure of the sound vibrations to be transmitted to the cochlea normally.

Volume

Air-borne sounds heard by an individual with normal hearing enter the external auditory canal and impinge upon the tympanic membrane; the membrane vibrates; the ossicles respond to these vibrations transmitting them into the cochlea. These physical vibrations are transformed into electrical impulses; the responses of the cochlear microphonics are transmitted by the eighth cranial nerve (auditory nerve) ultimately to the appropriate cerebral cortical areas and are recognized as sound.

Our environment is a relatively noisy one. An individual with normal hearing is constantly attuned to the changes of noise intensity about him. By adjusting the speech volume to the amounts of noise, we are able to achieve the proper volume alterations necessary to be heard above the ambient noise levels. Ruling out other influences of volume changes, the normal hearing person will adjust his volume satisfactorily.

Additionally, individuals with normal hearing hear their own voices by their own bone conduction. The normal hearing individual relies on this dual mechanism for monitoring the volume of his own speech: (1) normal air conduction conditioned by the ambient noise level, and (2) normal bone conduction relative to this.

A person with bilateral conductive deafness suffers from alterations of his speech volume because to such a patient the ambient noise may be minimal or non-existent, and he feels as though he is listening in a quiet, subdued, cathedral-like world. He will necessarily reduce his volume which he is monitoring by this artificially quiet environment.

The weak volume is further influenced by the *relatively* increased bone conductivity, as the patient is more aware of hearing by his own bone conduction than the normal hearing individual. In order to minimize his hearing of his own speech by his own bone conduction, he will make a further effort to reduce his volume.

In summary, his monitoring ceiling has been lowered both by the apparent reduced ambient noise of his own making and also by his relatively increased bone conduction.

Pitch

Pitch deviation is another speech defect noted in conductive deafness. Pitch, not to be confused with volume, refers to the position of an individual's voice on a musical scale (frequency of vibrations—cycles per second).

Anomalies of volume are described as being weak or excessive. Pitch deviations are described as being low, high and, possibly, monotonous.

The incidence of low pitch (key) and monotonous pitch pattern is very frequent with conductive deafness. The patient will reduce the volume of his voice so that it sounds satisfactory to himself. Pitch key, which is directly correlated with a volume change, will be lowered. The result is an over-relaxation of the vocal cords thus altering the physical characteristics of the cords (length, tension, and thickness) .

A reduction of volume and a lowering of pitch manifests itself in a general lack of pitch variation resulting in monotonous delivery of the speech. The speaker's lack of shifts, inflections and intonation give the listener the impression that the speaker is uninterested in what he has to say. Thus the listener, too, will often lose interest.

Quality

Quality as previously stated is pitch plus resonance. Musical instruments vary in quality due to the materials of the resonator (wood or metal) and the size and shape of the mouthpiece, string or reed. By the use of a mute on the musical instrument its quality can be changed further.

In the human "musical instrument" an alteration of the proper resonator will result in an aberration of phonation. With conductive deafness, the nasal sounds M, N, NG are subdued in the oral cavity instead of being reinforced in the nasal cavity, because of bone conduction already described. This speech deviation is termed *denasal quality.*

Sounds resonated in the nasal cavity will appear to sound louder to the speaker than those resonated in the mouth. The person with conductive deafness perceives his own bone-conducted phonations at greater intensity than those heard by air conduction. Sounds which produce a greater intensity because of the greater amount of bone stimulation, as do the nasal sounds, are incomparably loud. Unconsciously a nasopharyngeal seal is formed, preventing nasal sounds from entering the proper resonating cavity. These nasal sounds are now made as mouth sounds, resulting in a type of quality deviation frequently observed in individuals suffering from an acute rhinitis or nasal block. The phoneme M sounds like B; N sounds like D; and NG sounds like G.

Retracted quality is another speech deviation. For example, a ventriloquist is able to produce speech without moving his articulators by retracting his phonations. Our attention is held by the animated puppet and we are distracted from watching the ventriloquist himself. The speech sounds are made in the back of the throat and by "throwing his voice" he creates the illusion.

Speech sounds produced in the mouth strike the hard palate, the alveolus and the maxillae, thus setting the skull into vibration. Because of monitoring of speech hearing by bone conduction, the speaker is guided by his subjectivity and attempts to reduce the bone conduction. He pulls back or holds back the tongue, preventing the hard palate from vibrating vigorously. The speech sounds roll off the tongue and escape through the lips, resulting in minimal phonatory movements.

Articulation

Articulatory deviations are not as frequently apparent in the speech of persons with a conductive deafness, as in those with a perceptive loss of hearing. However, as moderate as these deviations are, they are recognizable as a deficiency.

The self hearing by bone conduction is the dominant factor in the monitoring of volume, pitch and quality of speech. This normal avenue of hearing is responsible also for the moderation of gross speech deviations in conductive deafness. The phonemes of M, N, NG when resonated in the nasal cavity (*see Quality*) sound subjectively too loud and the speaker attempts to guide these nasals into a cavity where they will not be manifested as too loud. The nasals are channeled into the oral cavity where the phonemes B, D,

G are substituted for the proper sounds. The sound of N may also be substituted for the NG sound.

Because the voiced consonant sounds are heard louder (apparently reinforced by bone conduction), unvoiced consonants which produce little or no vibrations of the skull are substituted for their voiced cognates. This occurs particularly when the voiced consonant is the final sound of a word rather than when it is in the initial or medial position of a word. For example, *had* becomes *hat, hands (z)* becomes *hands (s)*.

Weakening of consonants is another deviation associated with conductive deafness. The phonemes R and L when articulated correctly produce vigorous vibrations of the hard palate giving the patient the sensation of increased loudness. The phoneme R is weakened considerably and is replaced by W or a W-like sound substitution. The phoneme L is retracted and becames W or a W-like sound.

A diagnostic and therapeutic consideration for the preservation of speech sounds in the speech pattern is the visibility of the sound form as molded by the visible speech forming organs, such as the lips, teeth and tongue. Sounds whose forms or movements are invisible to the eye usually are substituted by a similar more visible sound. If the deafness has existed for a long period of time and the speaker has had to depend on speech (lip) reading, the invisible phonemes K, G, NG (sounds made in the back of the mouth) will be replaced by the more visible phonemes T, D, N. For example *car* becomes *tar, garage* becomes *darage,* and *hearing* becomes *hearin*.

Deviations of vowels and diphthongs are not as marked in conductive deafness as in perceptive deafness. However, as the volume of speech is reduced by the person with conductive impairment, there is also a reduction in the range of mobility of the articulators. Reduced volume imposes lessened movements of these organs and the function of the articulators becomes depressed and inactive. The speech is characterized by mumbling, general lack of precise articulation, dullness and flatness.

15

SPEECH DEVIATIONS IN PERCEPTIVE DEAFNESS

Perceptive deafness, nerve deafness, is the lack of sensitivity of the auditory mechanism in the cochlea; injury of the acoustic nerve, or its center in the brain.

Hard of Hearing Patients

Volume

Individuals with perceptive deafness in whom both air and bone thresholds are a horizontal curve over the range of frequencies will demonstrate an excessive amount of volume when they speak.

Let us assume that the cochlea is a harp-like organ. The strings on this harp vary in length, tension, and thickness. The resulting intensity of a particular string being plucked will depend on the pressure of the pluck. A light pluck might produce an intensity of 40 decibels, a heavier pluck one of 60 decibels. If some of the strings were to become loosened, a light pluck would produce a similar frequency but would produce a decreased intensity. In order to produce the original amount of intensity on this loosened string, it would now be necessary to increase the power of the pluck. In perceptive deafness, volume or pressure power may be compared with plucking power. The harp-like cochlea in the hearing mechanism has many loosened strings (frequency bands). Increase in volume or plucking power is necessary to allow the patient to hear his own volume at an acceptable level. Both exogenous and endogenous sounds are in need of reinforcement and this increase in volume is perceived as being of normal loudness.

In some patients the volume may be weak. Many of them demonstrate audiograms which slope from normal thresholds for the low frequencies to marked losses from the middle speech frequencies to the high frequencies. A male patient, because the phonatory pitch frequency falls in the lower registers, will monitor his volume within the range of his normal acoustic frequencies and tend to avoid those other pitches and frequencies which appear in his impaired hearing range. The volume of the female's voice with this type of loss will not demonstrate a diminution because her voice generally does not include the lower pitches. However, the volume of the female voice may be reduced when there is no marked loss of hearing in the higher pitch range but a loss in frequencies considered low.

Pitch

Another deviation of the voice in perceptive deafness is a change in key and intonation. Numerous psychological factors influence pitch changes. Some of these factors are indifference, disgust, boredom, worry, anger, bitterness, anxiety, fatigue and preoccupation. The listeners must be especially careful when relying upon pitch as the means of diagnosing a particular type of hearing loss. When psychological factors can be discounted, perceptive deafness generally manifests itself in a lack of pitch variation, monotony of tone, and in some instances a raising of the pitch (key).

Lack of pitch variation, monotony, occurs because the

speaker attempts to reproduce by his own speech, the qualities of the speech of others and his own speech as they sound to him. He is unable to hear the constant fluctuating changes, both minimal and subtle, which characterize proper voice habits. Hearing only occasional emphatic shifts, inflections and intonations, he begins to omit the requisites of normal speech. When the deafness is severe and long standing, the loss of pitch control is so pronounced, that he tends to misplace the emphasis of his own speech thus producing abnormal meanings, colors and effects.

An individual with a conductive deafness usually lowers the pitch (key) of his voice and also reduces the volume. In perceptive deafness the opposite occurs; there will be an increase in volume which automatically raises the pitch. These abnormal volume and pitch deviations may often mislead the listener. The high-pitch, strident, harsh, querulous voice fails to convey to the listener the true feelings of the speaker. The perceptive hard of hearing individual is unable to introduce into his own speech the delicate nuances which the listening audience needs, whereby the attitudes, intents and emotions of the speaker are interpreted. Speech values such as irony, sarcasm, or humor are less readily produced by such patients. Hypertension of the vocal chords, the result of increased tonus, may cause pathology of the cords and a permanent malfunction.

Perceptive deafness for high tones with relative normal hearing in the middle registers usually results in speech in a proper key or a lowered key. Persons so affected produce aberrations which are similar to the pitch pattern associated with a conductive loss of hearing.

Quality

The first noticeable change in the voice and speech pattern of patients demonstrating a perceptive deafness occurs in abnormal quality of voice, most commonly nasality and stridency. These qualities are rather reliable guides for recognizing perceptive deafness speech patterns.

As stated in the chapter on conductive deafness, the bony structure of the skull is an excellent conductor of an individual's own speech sounds. The person with perceptive deafness appreciates the reinforcement of speech vibrations by the osseous structure. Speech sounds resonated in the nasal cavity are strengthened because of the large amount of bone enclosing that area. The proper reinforcement of the nasal phonemes M, N, NG does not appear too loud or disturbing to the patient, rather, he prefers this. Vowels, diphthongs, and consonants which are resonated in the mouth, an area enclosed by fleshy walls, are not perceived by him as well as sounds normally resonated in the nasal cavity. In order to strengthen the weakly perceived sounds the patient tends to funnel all speech sounds into the nose by the non-closure of the nasopharyngeal seal. Thus, many of the oral sounds will filter into the nasal cavity to produce for him the desirable reinforcement of these weakly perceived phonemes. The result is marked nasal quality.

Nasality in perceptive deafness may vary from a limited to excessive amount (nasal twang) depending on the frequencies of the oral sounds which are nasalized.

If there is an increase in the pitch of the voice due to an increased tension of the vocal musculatures, the patient with perceptive deafness will demonstrate also a strident quality. Stridency is produced by a combination of increased volume, a raised key and nasal resonance. The resulting voice is harsh-sounding and shrill. Dissonant high overtones are also produced. The patient is unaware of the unpleasant quality because he, himself, cannot hear this nor his other speech changes.

Retracted or throaty quality may be demonstrated by the

perceptively hard of hearing patient. The hard quality of tone is generally produced by considerable constriction in the muscles of the throat. The retracted quality provides a more positive means of channeling normally produced mouth sounds into the nasal cavity with its osseous structure. The oral frontal sounds are reinforced in the nasal passage and appear normal to the patient.

Articulation

Since we learn to speak by hearing and imitating what we hear, an individual with a loss of hearing will imitate speech as it sounds to him, heard through his defective sensory receptor. If a bilateral perceptive loss of hearing occurs prior to speech maturation, articulation deviations will necessarily result. With long-standing perceptive deafness, the patient will gradually forget the normal articulation pattern and develop speech deteriorations. Should the loss of hearing increase with time, the articulation faults will necessarily become more pronounced and profound.

The factors which influence the distortion, retention and imagery of speech sounds in perceptive deafness include: loss of hearing that is greater in the high frequency range than the low frequency range; inadequate visibility of some speech sounds; limitations of the bony structure of the skull to transmit sounds and aid in perception; weak phonetic power of certain speech sounds; the fact that the low frequency speech sounds mask out high frequency sounds; high frequency components of tinnitus; the structure of the ear which may be such that it responds more efficiently and effectively to low frequency sounds than to high frequency sounds.

The sibilant consonants S, SH, CH, J, ZH are either distorted, substituted one for another, or completely omitted in speech typical of perceptive deafness. These sounds have important high frequency components (3200-8000 cycles). An appreciable loss of hearing in this range impairs the perception of these sounds and blocks their reproduction. These sibilants are affected by all the factors mentioned previously such as poor lip reading ability, bone conduction limitations, weak phonetic power, low sounds (vowels and consonants) masking out high frequency sounds, structural construction of the ear, and tinnitus.

The fricatives F, V, TH (voiced and unvoiced) are deviated and distorted by similar influences which affect the production of the sibilants previously discussed. The high frequency range and the low phonetic power of these speech sounds are particularly important factors in poor retention and production of these speech sounds. The F and voiceless TH sounds are the least powerful sounds in speech.

The sounds of R and L are generally classified as semi-vowel, vowel-like consonants. These sounds when articulated correctly are essentially invisible on the lips. They fall in the 2400 to 3000 cycle bands. Poor bone conductivity and high frequency sounds being masked out by the lows, usually give the perceptively deaf a distorted impression of these phonemes and produce defective reproductions.

The sounds of K and G are also characterized by faulty production or distortion. These speech sounds are classified as back-of-the-mouth sounds and have a low lip-reading ratio. If the deafness is of long duration the individual, therefore, fails to see and comprehend the K and G phonemes. Inevitably he will substitute in his own speech production the more visible similar frontal sounds T and D.

Vowel and diphthong distortion and confusion are another characteristic of speech in perceptive deafness. A flattening of the vowels occurs as the speaker attempts to go from weakly perceived consonants onto stronger perceived consonants. In his haste he passes over these vowels and diphthongs and also increases the rate of his speech. Many vowels and diphthongs having a low visibility factor in terms of speech (lip) reading are difficult to interpret purely from their lip positions.

Associated with the distorted production of the S sound, consonants clustered with the S phoneme will also be deviated (ST, TS, SK, KS, PS, and others). The high frequency components of these clusters also are factors in their poor production.

Speech Patterns of the Deafened

The degree of speech deviations demonstrated by the deafened individual will depend upon the following factors: *Age of onset.* Did the loss occur in early childhood or in proximity to the age of speech maturation or did it occur after the cerebral speech patterns were well established? *Duration of the deafness.* How long has the hearing loss existed? *Individual differences.* Some persons will suffer deterioration of speech and voice patterns more rapidly and more severely than others. *Previous training.* Were there any attempts to preserve or correct the speech deviations?

This deafness results in a rapid deterioration of voice and articulation, and in many instances there is a loss of speech intelligibility. Unrelated sounds such as audible breathing and grunts precede and succeed the phonation of words and phrases. The voice is retracted and lacks proper resonance. Volume is uncontrolled and often is loud. The excessive volume induces a strident quality. The pitch pattern is completely deviated and lacks normal shifts, inflections and intonations. The speech pattern is staccato and dull with an increase in rate. There is a general tendency to hurry over the vowels and clip short vowels and consonants.

Speech Patterns of the Deaf

Since this profound hearing loss develops prior to the patient's learning to speak, he is unable to produce sounds that he has never heard. He has no speech imagery or pattern to monitor. He has never heard humans engaged in conversation. Even after special schooling the newly learned speech patterns rarely approach the normal.

16

AUDITORY REHABILITATION

The goals of auditory rehabilitation are (1) to correct the motor and sensory communicative modalities, (2) to develop and utilize auditory, visual, and kinesthetic clues to attain maximum function, and (3) to teach the patient to learn to live with his handicap and overcome the effects of his disability.

Auditory rehabilitation includes both medical and surgical treatment and non-medical educational services. The individual's otorhinological structures are restored to as healthy and normal a state as possible. Many persons having a loss of hearing may never achieve normal hearing. Many, however, can be rehabilitated to resume their participation in adequate communication. The learning process can best be accomplished where there is trained staff and equipment to service, diagnose and treat hearing losses. This is the function of an auditory rehabilitation service.

Programs of auditory rehabilitation are designed to help individuals overcome the disorders of communication subsequent to impaired hearing and speech. Since these disorders often produce adverse changes in the attitudes of the patient toward society and of his fellow man toward him, the program seeks to furnish the patient the "tools" of communication. Its purpose is to help him understand the problems caused by his disability, to emphasize positive values, and to make use of his residual communication abilities.

The functions of a rehabilitation unit are to diagnose, to determine whether amplification is beneficial, to select the proper hearing aid, and to promote rehabilitative treatment. This type of treatment recognizes individual differences and limitations among the learners. Differences of intelligence and motivation, age, educational growth, vocational interests, environment, degrees of deafness, duration of the deafness, and the effect of the disability upon the individual are important considerations.

Obtaining a hearing aid for patients, training them in its use, and meeting their other communicative needs presents a formidable total audiological problem. In order to meet the needs these problems present, rehabilitation includes the following services:

Audiological Evaluation

(1) Otological history and examination.

(2) Hearing tests, including pure tone audiometry, speech audiometry, tests for psychogenic and simulated deafness, tolerance thresholds, and the ability to discriminate speech in the presence of noise.

(3) Psychological investigation when indicated.

(4) Speech and voice analysis including a permanent disc recording.

(5) Analysis of speech (lip) reading ability and auditory proficiency.

Auditory Rehabilitation

(1) Hearing aid selection.

(2) Fabrication of ear inserts.

(3) Instruction programs in speech (lip) reading (ele-

mentary and advanced), speech and voice correction, speech conservation, and auditory training.

(4) Orientation lectures on medical, psychological and vocational aspects of deafness.

(5) Individual and group psychological orientation and therapy as indicated.

Earlier chapters have presented the manifold investigations of persons with the symptom of impaired hearing. We are now prepared to enter an affirmative program of rehabilitation.

Speech (Lip) Reading

Speech (lip) reading is a method of understanding a speaker's verbalization by watching and interpreting the movements of his mouth, the expression in his eyes and his face, and his gestures. These visual clues must be supplemented by psychological clues of anticipation and synthesis.

Speech reading can provide assistance to those who have a sufficient loss of hearing regardless of the degree of the loss. The limitations of the hearing aid deny the user complete hearing under all conditions necessary for hearing and discriminating conversational speech. The frequency spectrum of many aids fails to include the highest speech frequencies effectively. Patients with perceptive deafness, with or without recruitment, and with discrimination losses do not receive the maximum potential improvement which an aid can yield. The gaps left by the hearing aid must be supplemented and filled in by visual clues. Effectiveness of a hearing aid is roughly inversely proportional to the kind and severity of the deafness. The most severely acoustically impaired patients can expect the least amount of acoustic serviceability from a hearing aid.

In some instances, speech reading serves the purpose of reinforcing the perception of speech while in other cases, as with the deaf and the deafened, speech reading is the only means of achieving an understanding even when speech is amplified by means of a hearing aid.

The teaching of speech (lip) reading can be accomplished both on an individual basis or as group therapy. These approaches are utilized according to the indications. A speech reading program should include a basic elementary speech reading course and an advanced speech reading course.

Basic or fundamental speech reading is designed to teach the acoustically handicapped individual to interpret speech without fully hearing it or, if necessary, without hearing it at all. The elementary course introduces speech sounds which are identified as either vowels or consonants, with each category defined and its purpose in connected speech explained. Further, the means of recognizing each is demonstrated and taught. For example, beginning with the consonants P, B, M, these sounds are made by the lips and revealed by the closure of the lips. Each of these phonemes is demonstrated in isolation so as to make the patient aware of how comparatively easily they can be seen and read. However, it is also demonstrated that these sound forms are identical visually. The phonemes P, B, M as in the words *pay, bay,* and *may,* cannot be identified by their visual clues and therefore must be distinguished by context.

Consonants are grouped homophonously and their production and revelation are demonstrated. Each group is further presented first in words, then in phrases and sentences, and finally used in longer passages. Each lesson is built about a basic unit of thought thus providing continuity and greater use of synthesis and association of ideas. Discussions evolving about current events, occupations, food, hobbies, television and movies, and newspaper stories are utilized. As the patient's speech reading ability increases, more material of greater complexity and abstraction is introduced.

Advanced speech reading is designed to develop speech reading ability of conversational efficiency. Practice material should provide for interpreting the speech of several individuals in rapid succession. Short plays, both with and without background sounds, intensive individual drill on vocabulary pertaining to the patient's vocational needs, and miscellaneous directed conversation are utilized.

Auditory Training

Auditory training teaches an individual to utilize his residual hearing more effectively. The effects of proper work done in auditory training are far-reaching. The aim is to improve the synthesizing ability of the patient, to train him to become an alert and discriminating listener with his hearing aid, to teach him to separate speech sounds so that they will become intelligible rather than a mass of jumbled noise, to develop tolerance for loud sounds, and to interpret speech in a noisy environment.

An auditory training program designed for many types of hearing losses is composed as follows:

(1) An explanation of the hearing aid fitting procedure with sample test material is presented to familiarize the patient with stimuli similar to those encountered during the fitting of the hearing aid.

(2) Discussions of the advantages and limitations of the hearing aid. Maximum and minimum benefits are explained.

(3) Discussion of the development of the electronic hearing aid. Care of the hearing aid, batteries and parts, gar-

ments, and reasons for occasional malfunction of the hearing
aid.

(4) Identification of gross sounds and classification (en-
joyment, environmental, and responses) with particular
attention to the importance of synthesis.

(5) Explanation of the audiogram-types of deafness and
kinds of audiometric curves. Explanation of each patient's
audiogram-relationship of speech sounds and their position
on the frequency spectrum.

(6) Speech discrimination word list, practice-lists of
short words containing identical vowels but different final
or initial consonants.

(7) Listening practice, explanation of types of listening
situations.

Easy listening. One voice, easy rate, clear diction, and
subdued background music.

Medium listening. Voice with choral background, words
running together, and regionalism.

Difficult listening. Fast rate, unexpected words, uncom-
mon words and ideas, foreign accent, group singing or
group speaking, unfamiliar ideas.

(8) Listening against a background of irrelevant noise.
This is done with and without lip reading (depending upon
severity and kind of deafness).

(9) Developing tolerance for loud sounds.

(10) Localization of source of sound or speech.

(11) Telephone technique, use of telephone with hearing aid and use of amplified telephones.

Another group consists of those adults whose deafness
originated in childhood, and who have never been given any
formal training in hearing, speaking and speech reading.
These patients should be offered the opportunity of rehabil-

itation, although the prognosis may not be as bright as with young children whose learning potential is enormous. Nevertheless, with long-term training these patients can learn to speak better and to lip read.

With the profound losses that these patients demonstrate, and presumably with the failure of adequate cerebral word imagery, amplification usually will not contribute to their adequate hearing and discriminating of speech. However, with amplification these patients can learn to recognize gross environmental sounds and recognize the human voice. These are large rewards in terms of the great deficit in acoustical intelligibility.

Hearing Aid Check List for Patients

(1) *Ear Insert*
  a. Keep free of wax.
  b. How to clean.

(2) *Receiver*
  a. When defective, results in weak and tinny reception.
  b. Considerations of feedback.

(3) *Cords*
  a. Awareness of polarity.
  b. Non-reversibility end for end.
  c. Intermittent operation when broken.

(4) *Transmitter*
  a. Care in handling.
  b. Do not get wet.
  c. Avoid extreme heat. Do not leave in closed car on hot day.

(5) *Batteries*
  a. Corrosion of battery terminal.
  b. Cleaning contacts in the aid.
  c. Proper tension at contact points.
  d. Know the end point voltage.
  e. Possibility of reversing battery when placing in aid.

Speech Conservation and Correction

Speech correction therapy in an auditory rehabilitation program is a program of therapy to correct and alleviate speech deviations. These deviations will disrupt either the entire speech pattern or particular areas. Speech defects depend upon many factors. These are the age of the patient, age of the onset of the hearing loss, type of deafness, and severity of the loss.

The following sample speech correction programs can be adapted to meet the individual speech needs subsequent to a loss of hearing:

(1) Thorough diagnosis of the voice and speech patterns of the patient by use of a formal speech examination. Prepared test sentences to help in the diagnosis of all deviated consonants, vowels, and diphthongs should be used. Deviations of volume, pitch, rate and voice quality should also be carefully noted.

(2) A recording of the patient's voice is made, eliciting conversational material for the recording either by outline or interview technique. The recording is then played back and the patient's speech and voice deviations are pointed out and demonstrated to him.

(3) Before any corrective work is begun, the physiology of the breathing and speech mechanism is explained.

(4) Speech conservation. This part of the program is designed as insurance against future deterioration of the voice and speech pattern. The relationship between a loss of hearing and its effect upon the normal speech pattern is discussed in order to acquaint the patient with all the probable reasons for these changes.

(5) Volume deviations are corrected and the patient's

voice is corrected to the appropriate level through the use of skits and plays, decibel meter and tape recordings.

(6) After volume control is learned, correction of faulty pitch pattern (key-inflection-intonation) is begun by the use of the piano, tuning forks and tape recorder.

(7) Voice quality deviations are discussed and demonstrated and corrective work is begun.

(8) Corrective work is done on speech rate problems as they arise. The patient is made aware of this deviation and practice drills are introduced.

(9) Final correction problem is one of specific consonant, vowel and diphthong deviations. Use is made of the multisensory approach including auditory stimulation, visual, motor-kinesthetic and tactile sensitivity. Drill of the faulty sound or sounds in isolation, initial, medial and final sounds in words, and in "loaded sentences" is done.

(10) At the conclusion of the speech program, a final recording is made. The original and final recordings are played for comparison.

BIBLIOGRAPHY

Chapters 1-10

Accepted Apparatus. Council on Physical Medicine and Rehabilitation, J.A.M.A. 1953.

A Guide for Conservation of Hearing in Industry.
American Academy of Ophthalmology and Otolaryngology. Subcommittee on Noise in Industry of the Committee on Conservation of Hearing. Los Angeles.

American Standard Acoustical Terminology, Z24.1 New York, American Standards Association, Inc. (ASA). 1951

Atkinson, M.: Tinnitus aurium, some considerations concerning its origin and treatment. A.M.A. Arch. Otolarygn. *45*:68, 1948.

Bergman, M.: The audiology clinic: A manual for planning a clinic for the rehabilitation of the acoustically handicapped. Acta oto-laryng., Supp. 89. 1950.

Bordley, J. E., and Hardy, W. G.: A study in objective audiometry with the use of a psychogalvanometric response. Ann. Otol., Rhin. & Laryng. *58*: 751-760, 1949.

Denes, P., and Naunton, R. E.: The clinical detection of auditory recruitment. J. Laryng. & Oto. *64*: 375-398, 1950.

Dix, M. R., and Hallpike, C. S.: Peep show—new technique for pure tone audiometry in young children. Brit M.J. *2:* 719-723, 1947.

Dix, M. R., Hallpike, C. S., and Hood, J. D.: Observations upon the loudness and recruitment phenomenon, with special reference to the differential diagnosis of disorders of the internal ear and VIII nerve. Proc. Roy. Soc. Med. *61*: 516-526, 1948.

211

Doerfler, L. G., and Stewart K.: Malingering and psychogenic deafness. J. Speech Disorders *11*: 181-186, 1946.

Eby, L. G., and Williams, H. L.: Recruitment of loudness in the differential diagnosis of end-organ and nerve fiber deafness. Laryngoscope *61*: 400-414, 1951.

Fletcher, H., and Munson, W. A.: Loudness, its definition, measurement and calculation. Jour. Acoust. Soc. Amer. *5*: 82-108, 1933.

Fowler, E. P.: Tests of hearing. In Medicine of the Ear. Fowler, E. P., Jr., Ed. New York, Thomas Nelson & Sons, 1939.

————: Tinnitus aurium in the light of recent research. Ann. Otol., Rhin. & Laryng. *50*:139, 1943.

————: The control of head noises, their illusion of loudness and timbre. A.M.A. Arch. Otolaryng. *37*: 391, 1943.

————: Tinnitus in normal and diseased ears. A.M.A. Arch. Otolaryng. *39*: 498, 1944.

————: Nonvibratory tinnitus, factors underlying subaudible and audible irritations. Transact. Am. Laryng., Rhin. & Otol. Society, 1947.

————: Emotional factors in tinnitus. Laryngoscope *58*: 145-154, 1948.

Fowler, E. P., Jr.: Medical aspects of hearing loss. In Hearing and deafness. H. David Ed. pp. 67-100. New York, Rinehart, 1947.

Harris, J. D.: An historical and critical review of loudness recruitment. New London, Conn: Naval Medical Research Laboratory, Report No. 200, Vol. XI, 1952.

————: Normal hearing and its relation to audiometry. Laryngoscope, *64*: 928-956, 1954.

Heller, M. F.: Audiology. New York Med. *7*: 16-17, 34-37, 1951.

————, and Bergman, M.: Tinnitus aurium in normal hearing persons. Ann. Otol., Rhin. & Laryng. *61*: 78-83, 1953.

————, and Lindenberg, P.: The private practice of auditory rehabilitation. Ann. Otol., Rhin. & Laryng. *63*:130, 1954.

——, and ——: Evaluation of deafness of non-organic origin. A.M.A. Arch. Otolaryng. *58*: 575-581, 1953.

Hirsh, I. J.: The measurements of hearing. New York, McGraw-Hill, 1952.

————, Palva, T., and Goodman, A.: Difference limen and recruitment. A.M.A. Arch. Otolaryng. *60:* 525-540, 1954.

Hudgins, C. V., Hawkins, J. E., and Karlin, J. E.: The development of recorded auditory tests for measuring hearing losses for speech. Laryngoscope *57*: 57-89, 1947.

———, and Ross, D. A.: The measurement of hearing. Volta Review, *49*: No. 3, 1947.

Jerger, J. F.: A difference limen recruitment test and its diagnostic significance. Laryngoscope, *62:* 1316-1332, 1952.

———: Difference limen difference test. A.M.A. Arch. Otolaryng. *57*: 490-500, 1953.

Kastein, S., and Fowler, E. P. Jr.: Differential diagnosis of communication disorders in children referred for hearing disorders. A.M.A. Arch. Otolaryng. *60*: 468-477, 1954.

Kerrison, P. D.: Disease of the ear, p. 130. Philadelphia, J. P. Lippincott, 1930.

Kopetzky, S. J.: Deafness, tinnitus, and vertigo, p. 153. New York, Thomas Nelson and Sons, 1948.

Lempert, J.: Tympano-sympathectomy, a surgical technic for the relief of tinnitus. A.M.A. Arch. Otolaryng. *43*:199, 1946.

Lüscher, E., and Zwislocki, S.: A simple method for indirect monaural determination of the recruitment phenomenon, difference limen in intensity in different types of deafness. Acta oto-larygn., Supp. *78*: 156-168, 1949.

Michels, M. W., and Randt, C. T.: Galvanic skin response in a differential diagnosis of deafness. A.M.A. Arch. Otolaryng. *45*: 302-311, 1947.

Priest, R. E.: Tests for unilateral deafness. A.M.A. Arch. Otolaryn. *42*: 138-143, 1945.

Reger, S. N.: Differences in loudness response of the normal and hard of hearing at intensity levels slightly above threshold. Ann. Otol., Rhin. & Laryng. *45*: 1029-1039, 1936.

Report on the Relations of Hearing Loss to Noise Exposure. Z24-X-2. New York, American Standards Association, Inc. (ASA), 1954.

Saltzman, M.: Clinical audiology. New York, Grune & Stratton, 1949.

Sonnenschein, R.: The nose, throat and ears and their diseases. Jackson, C. and Coates, G. M., Ed. pp. 472-491. Philadelphia, W. B. Saunders, 1930.

Stevens, S. S., and Davis, H.: Hearing. New York, John Wiley and Sons, 1947.

Utley, J.: Suggestive procedures for determining auditory acuity in very young acoustically handicapped children. Eye, Ear, Nose & Throat Monthly, *28*: 590-595, 1949.

Wegel, R. L.: A study of tinnitus. A.M.A. Arch. Otolaryng. *14*:158, 1931.

Chapters 11-12

Albrite, J. P.: The development and application of a soft ear mold, A.M.A. Arch. Otolaryng. *61*: 235-236, 1955.

————, and Glorig, A.: Modified soft ear insert, A.M.A. Arch. Otolaryng. *61*: 328-330, 1955.

Carhart, R.: Selection of hearing aids. Arch. Otolaryng. *44*: 1-18, 1946.

————: Tests for selection of hearing aids. Laryngoscope *56*: 780-794, 1947.

————: Hearing aid selection by university clinics. J. Speech & Hearing Disorders *15*: 106-113, 1950.

————: Speech audiometry in clinical evaluation. Acta oto-laryng. *41*: 18-42, 1952.

————, and Thompson, E.: The fitting of hearing aids. Tr. Am. Acad. Ophth. *51*: 354-361, 1947.

Corliss, E. L. R.: Hearing aids. Washington, D. C., U. S. National Bureau of Standards, Circular 534, 1953.

Davis, H.: Hearing Aids. *Hearing and deafness.* pp. 161-210. New York, Rinehart, 1947.

————: The articulation area and the social adequacy index for hearing. Laryngoscope *58*: 761-778, 1948.

————, et al: The selection of hearing aids. Laryngoscope *56*: 85-115, 135-163, 1946.

————, et al.: Hearing aids; An experimental study of design objectives. Cambridge, Harvard University Press, 1947.

Egan, J. P.: Articulation testing methods. Laryngoscope *58*: 955-991, 1948.

Fletcher, H.: A method of calculating hearing loss for speech from an audiogram. Acta oto-laryng., Supp. *90*: 26-37, 1950.

Harris, J. D.: Some suggestions for speech reception testing. Arch. Otolaryng. *50*: 388-405, 1949.

Hirsh, I. J., et al: Development of materials for speech audiometry. J. Speech and Hearing Disorders *17*: 321-337, 1952.

Hudgins, C. V., et al.: The development of recorded auditory tests for measuring hearing loss for speech. Laryngoscope *57*: 57-89, 1947.

Jeffers, J.: Quality judgment with respect to hearing aid selection. Ph.D. Thesis, Columbia University. 1955.

Johnson, K. O., and Newby, H. A.: Experimental study of the efficiency of two group hearing tests. Arch. Otolaryng. *60*: 702-710, 1954.

Lidén, G.: Speech Audiometry. Acta oto-laryng. Supp. *114*: 1-145, 1954.

————, and Fant, G.: Swedish word material for speech audiometry and articulation tests. Acta oto-laryng., Suppl. *116*: 189-204, 1954.

Nichols, R. H., Jr.: Physical characteristics of hearing aids. Laryngoscope, *57*: 31-40, 1947.

Palva, T.: Finnish speech audiometry. Acta oto-laryng., Suppl. *101*: 1-128, 1952.

Silverman, S. R.: Use of speech tests for evaluation of clinical procedures. Arch. Otolaryng. *51*: 786-797, 1950.

Silverman, S. R., and Taylor, G.: The choice and use of hearing aids. *Hearing and Deafness,* pp. 211-254. Ed. by H. Davis. New York, Rinehart, 1947.

Watson, L. A., and Tolan, T.: The modern hearing aid. *Hearing tests and hearing instruments,* pp. 268-347. Baltimore, Williams & Wilkins, 1949.

Chapters 13-16

Anderson, V.: Training the speaking voice. New York, Oxford University Press, 1942.

Ansberry, M.: Rehabilitation of the deaf and hard of hearing, pp. 29-32. Washington, D. C., Federal Security Agency, Office of Vocational Rehabilitation, 1950.

Avery, E., Dorsey, J., and Sickles, V.: First principles of speech training. New York, D. Appleton, Century, 1930.

Berry, M., and Eisenson, J.: The defective in speech. New York, Crofts, 1945.

Brentano, L.: Ways to better hearing. New York, Franklin Watts, 1946.

Carhart, R.: Hearing deficiencies and speech problems. J. Speech Disorders, *8*: 247-254, 1943.

Davis, H.: Hearing and deafness. New York, Rinehart, 1947.

Ewing, I., and Ewing, A.: The handicap of deafness. New York, Longmans, Green, 1946.

Fletcher, H.: Speech and hearing. New York, Van Nostrand, 1929.

Jackson, C., and Jackson, C. L.: Diseases of the nose, throat and ear, p. 513, Philadelphia, W. B. Saunders, 1946.

Newhart, H.: Hearing deficiencies in relation to speech defects. Laryngoscope *48*: 129-136, 1938.

Pauls, M., Haskins, H., and Hardy, W. G.: Hearing and speech rehabilitation; speech reading, auditory rehabilitation and speech correction in re-education program. U. S. Nav. Med. Bull. (Supp.): 232-248, 1948.

Penn, J.: Hearing defects as factors influencing voice and speech patterns. Thesis, New York University, 1952.

Raubicheck, L.: How to teach good speech in the elementary schools. New York, Noble and Noble, 1937.

Van Riper, C.: Speech correction. New York, Prentice-Hall, 1937.

Watson, L., and Tolan, T.: Hearing tests and hearing instruments. Baltimore, Williams & Wilkins, 1949.

West, R., Kennedy, L., Carr, A., and Backus, O.: The rehabilitation of speech. New York, Harper & Bros., 1947.

INDEX

A

Ambient noise, 1, 4, 5, 172, 186, 187
American Schools for the Deaf
 Certifications, 8
American Speech and Hearing Association (A.S.H.A.)
 Certifications, 7-8
Amplifier
 carbon, 150
 vacuum-tube, 17, 21, 22, 29
Aphonia, hysterical or psychosomatic,
 185
Articulation
 deviations of,
  in conductive deafness, 190-192
  in perceptive deafness, 197-198
 site of, of consonants, 179-180
Astereophonia, 33-34, 86
Atkinson, M., 105
Attenuator, 17-18
Audible friction
 absence of, in vowels, 181
 in consonants, 179-180
Audiogram
 air conduction, 58, 87
 bone conduction, 58
 in non-organic deafness, 87, 89
 pure tone
  examples, 59-61
  and relation to speech tests, 131-
  147

standard symbols, 55-58
 See also Audiometers; Audiometry
Audiologic supplies, 29-30
Audiologic testing equipment
 list of, 29-30
 See also Testing equipment
Audiology centers, 6-13
 functions of, 6-7
 minimum equipment in, 10-11
 patient evaluation at, 12
 personnel of, 7-9, 12
 physical facilities of, 9-10
 services of, 7, 11-13
 standards for, 6
Audiometers, 14-18, 20, 24
 clinical, 11, 15, 79
 discrete frequency, 15-16
 internal design of, 17
 pure tone, 11, 14, 29, 119, 120
 single channel, 18, 67, 72
 sweep frequency, 15-16, 53
 two-channel, 10, 11, 14, 18, 67, 72
 Western Electric, 119
 See also Audiogram; Audiometry
Audiometry
 calibration, 17, 21, 55, 125-129
 for children, 113-117
  peep show, 2, 24-26, 64
  psychogalvanic skin test, 114-115
 conditioning in, 62-64
 pure tone, 2, 11, 14, 45-64, 92-93,
  113
  air conduction, 47-48

217